HEADACHE

CONTEMPORARY PATIENT MANAGEMENT SERIES

HEADACHE

Seymour Diamond, M.D.
Director, Diamond Headache Clinic
Adjunct Associate Professor of Pharmacology
The Chicago Medical School
Chicago, Illinois

Arnold P. Friedman, M.D.
Consultant, Neurological Associates of Tucson
Adjunct Professor of Clinical Neurology
University of Arizona Medical School
Tucson, Arizona

MEDICAL EXAMINATION PUBLISHING CO., INC.
an Excerpta Medica company

Diamond, Seymour, (date)
    Headache.

    Bibliography: p.
    Includes index.
    1. Headache. I. Friedman, Arnold P. II. Title.
RC392.D497   1983   617'.51   83-12188
ISBN 0-87488-892-1

Copyright © 1983 by
MEDICAL EXAMINATION PUBLISHING CO., INC.
an Excerpta Medica company
3003 New Hyde Park Road
New Hyde Park, New York

Printed in the United States of America

This book is dedicated to

Elaine Diamond and Sara Friedman

Contents

Preface

There have been many extensive texts on headache treatment, diagnosis and management. However, in this maze of books, few have been of any practical value for the average physician. With this factor in mind, the authors have endeavored to present a concise, easily applicable technique in the management of the headache patient.

Headache is probably one of the most frequent complaints for which a patient will consult a physician. It is also probably the most ignored complaint and most inconsistently treated condition. In this book an attempt has been made to coordinate an understandable approach to the many headache problems.

Acknowledgments

We would like to thank the following for their assistance in the completion of this book:

Joseph C. Battista, M.D., Department of Surgery, Medical College of Wisconsin, Affiliated Hospitals, Milwaukee, Wisconsin

Merle Diamond, M.D., Department of Internal Medicine, Section of Emergency Medicine, Northwestern Memorial Hospitals, Chicago, Illinois

Mary Franklin Epstein, R.N., Diamond Headache Clinic, Chicago, Illinois

Ned Mogabgab, M.D., Department of Internal Medicine, Section of Emergency Medicine, Northwestern Memorial Hospitals, Chicago, Illinois

notice

The authors and the publisher of this book have made every
effort to ensure that all therapeutic modalities that are recommended are in accordance with accepted standards at the time
of publication.

The drugs specified within this book may not have specific
approval from the Food and Drug Administration in regard to
the indications and dosages that may be recommended by the
authors. The manufacturer's package insert is the best source
of current prescribing information.

Chapter 1

Classification and Mechanism of Headache

A simple classification divides headaches into three main groups, based on the mechanism by which the pain is produced: (1) vascular headaches, which include headaches caused by abnormal reaction of the cerebral arteries, particularly a tendency toward dilatation; (2) muscle contraction (tension) headaches, produced by persistent contraction of the muscles of the head, neck, and face; and (3) traction and inflammatory headaches, which include all headaches secondary to organic disease of the skull and its components. There is also a fourth group: (4) idiopathic cranial neuralgias, in which no pathologic changes are found.

About 8% of headache patients seen by the generalist and over 50% of those seen by a headache specialist or in a pain clinic have vascular headaches. The primary examples of vascular headache are migraine and cluster. In the classic form of migraine, focal neurologic symptoms precede or, less often, accompany the headache; in so-called common migraine, the focal neurologic symptoms are absent. Depending on the most prominent focal symptom, more specific forms of migraine, although relatively rare, can be identified: ophthalmic, basilar artery, ophthalmoplegic, or hemiplegic. When the focal neurologic deficit persists longer than the headache, the migraine is known as "complicated" migraine. In some forms of migraine, whether classic or common, the pain is located atypically—in the face (facial migraine) or the cervical portion of the carotid artery (carotidynia). Still other types of migraine are characterized by specific patterns of recurrence, as in "weekend migraine" or "menstrual migraine".

Cluster headaches are so named because the attacks occur in groups, sometimes several per day over a period of weeks or months, after which the headaches then disappear, only to recur years later. Some unfortunate patients have unremitting

1

headaches.   Most authorities consider cluster headache a
variant of migraine, but others do not.

Muscle contraction headache is the most common type of headache seen by the family physician, and it is usually related to
stress, emotional conflicts, fatigue, or repressed hostility,
problems that may not be evident to the patient.   Chronic
muscle contraction headaches are often, although not exclusively,
associated with depression or anxiety.

Traction and inflammatory headache may be caused by cerebrovascular disease (stroke, hypertension, hemorrhage from an
aneurysm or arteriovenous malformation), brain tumor,
changes in intracranial pressure, infections, or inflammation.
The pain is produced by involvement of more than one pain-
sensitive structure, and the clinical profiles of these headaches
are varied.

The most common type of idiopathic cranial neuralgia is trigeminal neuralgia, which affects the branches of the fifth
cranial nerve.

In 1962, the National Institute of Neurological Diseases and
Blindness authorized a committee to prepare a classification
of headache.   It was published in JAMA, vol. 169, March 3,
1962, pp. 717-18.   The classification by the Ad Hoc Committee
was as follows:

Classification

1.   Vascular headaches of migraine type.   Recurrent attacks
     of headache, widely varied in intensity, frequency, and
     duration.   The attacks are commonly unilateral in onset;
     are usually associated with anorexia and, sometimes,
     with nausea and vomiting; in some are preceded by, or
     associated with, conspicuous sensory, motor, and mood
     disturbances; and are often familial.

     Evidence supports the view that cranial arterial distention
     and dilatation are importantly implicated in the painful
     phase but cause no permanent changes in the involved
     vessel.   Listed below are particular varieties of headache,
     each sharing some, but not necessarily all, of the above-
     mentioned features:

     A.   "Classic" migraine.   Vascular headache with sharply
          defined, transient visual and other sensory or motor
          prodromes or both.

B. "Common" migraine. Vascular headache without striking prodromes and less often unilateral than A and C. Synonyms are "atypical migraine" or "sick" headache. Calling attention to certain relationships of this type of headache to environmental, occupational, menstrual, or other variables are such terms as "summer," "Monday," "weekend," "relaxation," "premenstrual," and "menstrual" headache.

C. "Cluster" headache. Vascular headache, predominantly unilateral on the same side, usually associated with flushing, sweating, rhinorrhea, and increased lacrimation; brief in duration and usually occurring in closely packed groups separated by long remissions. Identical or closely allied are: ciliary or migrainous neuralgia (Harris), erythromelalgia of the head or histaminic cephalgia (Horton), and petrosal neuralgia (Gardner et al.).

D. "Hemiplegic" migraine and "ophthalmoplegic" migraine. Vascular headache featured by sensory and motor phenomena which persist during and after the headache.

E. "Lower-half" headache. Headache of possibly vascular mechanism, centered primarily in the lower face. In this group there may be some instances of "atypical facial" neuralgia, sphenopalatine ganglion neuralgia (Sluder), and vidian neuralgia (Vail).

2. Muscle contraction headache. Ache or sensations of tightness, pressure, or constriction, widely varied in intensity, frequency, and duration, sometimes long-lasting, and commonly suboccipital. It is associated with sustained contraction of skeletal muscles in the absence of permanent structural change, usually as part of the individual's reaction during life stress. The ambiguous and unsatisfactory terms "tension," "psychogenic," and "nervous" headache refer largely to this group.

3. Combined headache: vascular and muscle contraction. Combinations of vascular headache of the migraine type and muscle contraction headache prominently coexisting in an attack.

4. Headache of nasal vasomotor reaction. Headaches and nasal discomfort (nasal obstruction, rhinorrhea, tightness, or burning), recurrent and resulting from congestion and

edema of nasal and paranasal mucous membranes, and not proven to be due to allergens, infectious agents, or local gross anatomic defects. The headache is predominantly anterior in location, and mild or moderate in intensity. The illness is usually part of the individual's reaction during stress. This is often called "vasomotor rhinitis."

5.   Headache of delusional, conversion, or hypochondriacal states. Headaches of illnesses in which the prevailing clinical disorder is a delusional or a conversion reaction and a peripheral pain mechanism is nonexistent. Closely allied are the hypochondriacal reactions in which the peripheral disturbances relevant to headache are minimal. These also have been called "psychogenic" headaches.

N. B. The foregoing represent the major clinical disorders dominated by headache— those which are particularly common and in which headache is frequently recurrent and disabling.

6.   Nonmigrainous vascular headaches. These are associated with generally nonrecurrent dilatation of cranial arteries:

A.   Systemic infections, usually with fever.

B.   Miscellaneous disorders, including: hypoxic states; carbon monoxide poisoning; effects of nitrites, nitrates, and other chemical agents with vasodilator properties; caffeine withdrawal reaction; circulatory insufficiency in the brain (in certain circumstances); postconcussion reactions; postconvulsive states; "hangover" reactions; foreign protein reactions; hypoglycemia; hypercapnia; acute pressor reactions (abrupt elevation of blood pressure, as with paraplegia or pheochromocytoma); and certain instances of essential arterial hypertension (e. g. , those with early morning headache).

7.   Traction headache. Headaches resulting from traction on intracranial vascular structures, by masses:

A.   Primary or metastatic tumors of meninges, vessels, or brain.

B.   Hematomas (epidural, subdural, or parenchymal).

C.   Abscesses (epidural, subdural, or parenchymal).

    D.   Postlumbar puncture headache ("leakage" headache).

    E.   Pseudotumor cerebri and various causes of brain swelling.

8. Headache due to overt cranial inflammation. Headaches due to readily recognized inflammation of cranial struc- tures, resulting from usually nonrecurrent inflammation, sterile or infectious.

    A.   Intracranial disorders: infections, chemical, or allergic meningitis; subarachnoid hemmorhage; postpneumoencephalographic reaction; arteritis; and phlebitis.

    B.   Extracranial disorders: arteritis and cellulitis.

Headache due to disease of ocular, aural, nasal and sinusal, dental, or other cranial or neck structures:

9. Headache due to spread of effects of noxious stimulation of ocular structures (as by increased intraocular pressure excessive contraction of ocular muscles, trauma, new growth, or inflammation).

10. Headache due to spread of effects of noxious stimulation of aural structure (as by trauma, new growth, or inflammation).

11. Headache due to spread of effects of noxious stimulation of nasal and sinusal structures (as by trauma, new growth, inflammation, or allergens).

12. Headache due to spread of effects of noxious stimulation of dental structures (as by trauma, new growth or inflammation).

13. Headache due to spread of pain from noxious stimulation of other structures of the cranium and neck (periosteum, joint, ligaments, muscles, or cervical roots).

14. Cranial neuritides. Caused by trauma, new growth, or inflammation.

15. Cranial neuralgias. Trigeminal (tic douloureux) and glossopharyngeal. The pains are lancinating ("jabbing"), usually in rapid succession for several minutes or longer, are limited to a portion or all of the domain

of the affected nerve, and are often triggered by end-organ stimulation.   Trigeminal neuralgia must be distinguished, in particular, from cluster headache (1,C), with which it is often confused.

N.B. So-called chronic post-traumatic headache may rise from any one of several mechanisms. Such headaches may represent sustained muscle contraction (2), recurrent vascular dilation (1, B), or rarely, local scalp or nuchal injury (13). In some patients, the post-traumatic pain is part of a clinical disorder characterized by delusional, conversion, or hypo-chondriacal reactions (5).

Headache diagnostic guide

Headache type	Frequency	Duration	Onset	Pain area	Characteristic pain	Associated symptoms	Signs	Triggers	Sex distribution
Migraine	Usually no more than 1/week; 1-2/month, typical	3 hours-3 days; typically 12-18 hours	Gradual	Unilateral: may switch sides or become bilateral	Throbbing, moderate to severe	Systemic—usually nausea or vomiting; visual aura in classic, no aura in common	Usually none	Stress, menstruation, alcohol, food additives	3:1 female
Cluster	1-3/day	30-90 minutes	Sudden; reaches peak intensity in 1-3 minutes	Unilateral, usually retro-orbital	Steady, severe	Usually none	Tearing; complete or partial Horner's syndrome	Reliably triggered by alcohol	10:1 male
Muscle contraction	1/week—virtually continuous	Usually 8-12 hours	Gradual	"Hatband"	Steady, dull	None	None	Stress	Equal distribution
Mass lesion	Varied	Varied	Varied, though onset of complaint may have been recent	Unilateral	Varied	Varied	May be focal neurologic	None known	Equal distribution
Psychogenic	Omnipresent	Omnipresent		Varied, but may be bilateral	Described as severe by patient but without corresponding behavior	Usually none	None	None	Equal distribution

Chapter 2

A Headache History: "The Key to Diagnosis"

The clinician's most valuable diagnostic tool is usually a detailed history. For headache patients, this is especially true, since most headaches have some emotional basis, and physical and neurological examinations of these patients are usually normal.

The history must be taken with genuine interest and concern, so that the patient will feel encouraged to ventilate his problems. For many headache patients, there is a genuine fear of a brain tumor or other catastrophic illness, and the history may be distorted or certain points may be omitted. Anxiety may damage the physician-patient relationship, and computerized forms will not produce a true history.

To enable the physician to identify the kinds of headaches present, the history should be short and concise. Certain points should be included in all headache histories. The following will outline these points and discuss the rationale for including them in the headache history.

Types of Headache

Since many patients suffer from more than one type of headache, it is essential to elicit from the patient how many types of headaches the patient can identify. Quite often, a patient with a long history of recurrent one-sided severe headaches will develop a daily constant headache. This may also be accompanied by a sleep disturbance, which is typical of depression.

Onset

In order to determine the type of headache, it is important to determine the age at which the headache initially started. Vascular headaches usually begin in childhood, adolescence, or the third and fourth decades. Those headaches which start in the fifth decade will usually have a psychogenic component, such as depression, but organic disease must be ruled out.

Determining the length of the illness is also important. A patient who notes a 10- to 40-year history of headache will usually not be suffering from an organic illness. A sudden onset of the headache with other neurological symptoms will alert the physician to a possible organic cause and be indicative that further testing is required.

Precipitating factors should also be discussed. Headaches following a trauma will also require further evaluation. The female may note that the headaches started about the time of her menarche or may be related to pregnancy or menopause.

Location

The site of the pain is essential in identifying the type of headache. Pain always localized on one side can be indicative of migraine or organic disease, unless the clinical features are typical of cluster headache, tic douloureux, or local changes in the eyes, sinuses, skull, or scalp. Generalized pain may indicate psychogenic components if there is no evidence of increased intracranial pressure. If the pain is localized to the eye alone, the physician should be suspicious of cluster headache or ocular disease. The "hatband" distribution of head pain is typical of headaches with psychogenic components. It is also important to note that migraine will switch sides.

Timing

In cluster headache, the patient will often complain of a headache which will awaken him in the middle of the night and will continue for a few minutes to a few hours. The headache associated with hypertension is typically present on awakening and disappears as the day continues. In contrast, sinus headache starts gradually in the morning and will increase in severity as the day progresses.

Frequency

Migraine occurs periodically, possibly once every one to two months. During pregnancy and vacations, migraine is often absent. However, many patients will complain of their headaches exclusively during vacations or on weekends. Cluster headaches are so named because of their occurrence in a series, lasting several weeks or months. These series most often appear in spring or fall. Occasionally, a patient with cluster headaches will complain of a chronic cluster headache. Muscle contraction headaches, seen by the headache clinician, are chronic in nature, and usually occur on a daily basis. Physical and neurological examinations on these patients are usually normal and do not confirm the diagnosis of a headache with a psychogenic origin.

Duration, Severity, and Character

The pain of the headache due to an organic cause is usually persistent and progressively increases in intensity. Migraine headaches will continue from 6 hours to 3 days or longer. The pain will not be a constant ache, but rather intense pulsating or throbbing. Cluster headache will also be throbbing, but is usually very severe and is described as deep and boring. The duration of cluster headache is short, lasting from several minutes to 3 to 4 hours. A shock-like, stabbing pain is present in tic douloureux and is typically neuritic in character, and will last from only 1 to 15 minutes. Persistent, dull, and nagging pain is typical of headaches due to a psychogenic component, and the pain will increase occasionally.

Prodromata

These warning symptoms are typical of classical migraine, and will usually occur 30 to 60 minutes preheadache. The symptoms are most often visual in nature, such as zigzag flashing lights and colors, scotomata, or hemianopia. It is believed that these symptoms originate in the visual cortex portions of the occipital lobe. Other prodromata include: strange odors, sensory phenomena such as paresthesias or hypothesias, vertigo, defects of mobility or coordination, oculomotor paralysis, or hemiparesis.

The visual disturbances may also occur with tumors or vascular disorders, such as an angioma. In some headache patients, as they grow older, the headache may diminish but the prodromata will continue to occur, without any headache following the visual symptoms.

Associated Symptoms

Migraine headaches are most often associated with nausea and vomiting. This is the reason migraine is described as a "sick headache. " Other associated symptoms include: phonophobia, photophobia, blurred vision, dizziness, ringing in the ears, and focal neurologic changes. Patients with cluster headache will complain of facial flushing, lacrimination, and a nasal discharge associated with their headaches. These symptoms often occur on the same side as the headache. If a patient complains of double vision, convulsions, or tinnitus, an organic cause of the headache should be ruled out. Patients suffering from headaches with a psychogenic component will have long lists of various somatic, emotional, and psychic symptoms.

Precipitating Factors

Many factors can precipitate migraine attacks, including: fatigue, stress, menstruation, ovulation, lack of sleep, bright sunlight, too much sleep, alcohol, and change in weather and barometric pressure. Foods containing tyramine or sodium nitrite can be causative factors. In the Chinese restaurant syndrome, monosodium glutamate can cause a vascularlike headache. It is common for migraine sufferers to create an environment impossible to handle. The stress resulting from this situation may trigger a headache. Drugs containing vasoactive materials may also induce a migraine.

Frequently, migraine first appears at the onset of menses. During pregnancy, migraine will disappear by the third month, but will reappear following the delivery of the child. Migraine often disappears with menopause. However, migraine may be prolonged if postmenopausal hormones are administered. In contrast, sometimes migraine which reappears at the time of menopause may be improved with the administration of estrogen therapy.

Headaches may be precipitated by the occupation of the sufferer. Munitions workers are exposed to nitrates, which cause vasodilation of the cerebral vessels and will resemble vascular headaches. Workers in poorly ventilated areas, such as mechanics, are exposed to carbon monoxide, which can trigger headaches. Headaches precipitated by exertion, such as straining or cough, are not always associated with intracranial tumors, and can often be benign. These benign exertional headaches can occur in conjunction with vascular headaches in some sufferers.

Sleep Pattern

A psychogenic factor in headaches is often determined by a sleep disturbance. Frequent awakening during the night and early awakening in the morning for no apparent reason is usually associated with depression. The anxious patient will often complain of difficulty falling asleep. Occasionally, an acute migraine attack will awaken a patient, but migraine is usually relieved by sleep. Cluster headaches often awaken patients from a sound sleep. Hypertensive headaches (over 210 mmHg/110 mmHg) usually present on awakening and disappear after the patient is up and about. Headaches associated with frontal sinusitis may commence early in the morning.

Emotional Factors

An inventory of emotional factors is essential in determining the psychological background of the headache sufferer. The patient should be carefully questioned regarding marital and family relationships; occupational, social, and environmental stresses; and any sexual difficulties. This discussion may allow the patient to ventilate any possible problems which would relate to his headaches. Since some patients will not communicate problems until they have become confident with the interviewer, the questioning may need to be repeated on follow-up visits.

Family History

Patients with migraine and depressive headaches will often present a family history of headaches. Most headache experts throughout the world concur that migraine is a hereditary disease.

Medical History

Prior history of head trauma may be presented during the questioning of the patient's medical history. The patient may reveal a prior history of convulsions associated with headaches and neck stiffness which may be indicative of cerebral vascular malformation, such as an angioma and so on. The patient's previous medical history may also determine the therapy for the headache problem—for example, propranolol is contraindicated in patients with asthma.

Surgical History

Prior surgery on a melanoma or other tumor may indicate that the tumor has metastasized to the brain and is triggering the headache. Obviously, history of any previous neurological surgery will alert the physician to rule out an organic cause of the headache. Previous spinal puncture may also be related to the headache problem.

Allergy

Headache symptoms may be exacerbated or intensified in patients with seasonal allergies during the allergy season.   However, no one has identified a specific antibody-antigen relationship to migraine.

Medications

Previous

If previous therapy with ergotamine therapy has helped the patient, the most likely diagnosis is migraine. Also, if antidepressants have been effective, depression is indicated. Therefore, it is essential that a careful inventory of medications taken previously as well as their results should be included in the history.

Current

Obviously, the physician should be aware of the medications the patient is currently taking for headaches and other indications. For example, reserpine used in hypertension therapy may precipitate or increase the severity of migraine attacks. Oral contraceptive, postmenopausal hormones, and the nitrates used in coronary artery disease may induce migraine in susceptible patients (see Chapter 13).

Psychotherapy

Treatment of psychological aspects is paramount because emotional factors can frequently precipitate a headache attack. The supportive doctor-patient relationship during the initial phase of therapy is a key step in treatment. The patient who beleives that the physician is really an interested, understanding, and sympathetic person will gain confidence, and it will then be possible to explore those factors in the patient's life situation that have led to resentment, hostility, self-punishment, and so forth. If allowed free expression of conflicts, resentments, and dissatisfactions, the patient will gain insight into how these emotional factors relate to the physiological basis of their headache attacks. The patient needs reassurance, support, and guidance in redirecting behavior patterns to deal more effectively and realistically with all major problems.

Drugs Which Can Serve as Provocative Factors in Headache

Nitrates
Indomethacin (Indocin)
Oral progestational medications
Oral vasodilators
Vitamin B_2
Nicotinic acid

Drugs Which, If Withdrawn, May Serve as Provocative
Factors in Headache

Ergot
Caffeine
Amphetamines
Many phenothiazines

Environmental stress at home, at work, or in social situations may bring about more tension or anxiety than the patient can endure. One of the first steps, greatly aided by the confidence engendered by the physician-patient relationship, is to remove as much adverse stress as possible from the patient's environment. This alone will most likely decrease the number of headache attacks.

The role of physician should be limited to supportive therapy, guidance, counseling, and situation insight. Interpretive analysis, uncovering transference, and long-term intensive therapy should be done only by the psychiatrist.

General Guidelines

The reader is referred to the accompanying flowchart as a guide to differential diagnosis.

DIFFERENTIAL DIAGNOSIS: HEADACHE

(Decision points in heavy outline)

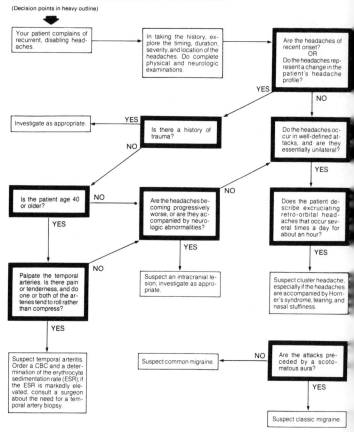

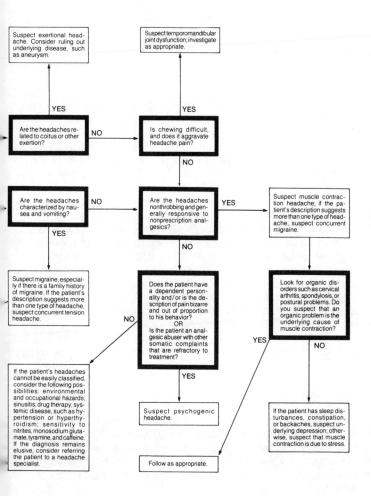

Chapter 3

Physical and Neurological Examination of the Headache Patient

---

A carefully detailed headache history should enable the physician to make an adequate diagnosis of the headache problem and rule out organic etiology. A thorough physical and neurological examination is also essential in order to determine which diagnostic tests will be necessary to confirm or rule out organic pathology. Certain items of particular relevance to headache should be checked.

During the history taking, much information may be gleaned by simply observing the patient. A person with a severe headache, whether it is organic or vascular, will usually walk and move quite slowly and deliberately, so as to avoid the jarring associated with walking which often intensifies the pain. The person who appears quite calm and relaxed but complains of severe, disabling headaches may have a headache in which psychogenic factors play an important part. Migraine sufferers often appear well-groomed and neat between attacks.

Blotching of the skin on the chest, sweaty palms, and occasionally, urticaria are evidence of the vasomotor instability of migraine.

Physical Examination

Determining the etiology of headaches may be aided by the vital signs. Fever of any cause is often accompanied by headache and should alert the physician to check for systemic disease or infection. One should rule out central nervous system infection, such as meningitis or abscess. Low-grade fever is often present in temporal arteritis.

Hypertension can produce a headache with typical features, but the diastolic pressure usually must be within the range of 120 to 140 mmHg or higher. Chronic vascular headaches may be increased in frequency and severity by just a mild blood pressure elevation. Although a diastolic pressure of 100 to 110 mmHg will not produce a headache by itself, it can aggravate a migraine attack. If the patient is quite tense, his pulse may be very rapid. A rapid pulse is also indicative of vasomotor lability.

After determining the vital signs, the physician should carefully inspect the head and examine it by palpation and auscultation. In patients with temporal arteritis or those in the middle of an acute migraine attack, the superficial temporal arteries may be quite prominent. Weakness due to a lesion of the seventh cranial nerve may cause an asymmetry of the face. It has been reported that patients with longstanding cluster headache have distinctive facial features: thick facial skin with deep furrows in the forehead and glabella, pitted coarse skin on the cheeks (peau d'orange), leonine facies, and telangiectasia on the nose and cheeks.

The eyes should be examined closely. During a headache attack, lacrimation and injection of the sclerae may be observed. Unilateral ptosis of the eyelid may occur in migraine or more often in cluster headache, and may continue for one to two days after the headache has subsided. If the ptosis continues between headache attacks, a tumor or aneurysm should be ruled out.

During examination, gross defects of the visual fields should be determined. The procedure includes the patient covering one eye and the examiner comparing the remaining visual field with his own range of vision by having the patient look directly at the examiner's face. The examiner then moves an object into the field of vision, such as a finger, pin, or light. The procedure is repeated with the other eye covered. If the patient has a possible loss of the full visual field or is complaining of visual symptoms which are not associated with the headache attack, a consultation with an ophthalmologist is indicated. Examination of the eyes is significant in the evaluation of the headache patient.

To evaluate intraocular tension, the eyeball should be palpated gently through the closed lid. Formal tonometry should be performed on patients with suspicious increased pressure. Testing extraocular eye movements in all directions is necessary to determine any weakness or the presence or absence of nystagmus. During examination, the optic fundi should be checked for papilledema and the presence or absence of venous pulsations. Increased intracranial pressure may be considered if the venous pulsations are absent at the disc margins. Other signs of increased intracranial pressure are hemorrhages or exudates in the retina in the absence of a blood dyscrasia, hypertension, or diabetes.

The nose should be examined for evidence of obstruction and
irritation.   A chronic low-grade headache may be caused by
vasomotor rhinitis with red, inflamed mucous membranes. Allergic rhinitis is indicated by swollen, edematous, and pale
mucosa.   Acute sinusitis will trigger a headache but is accompanied by fever and a purulent nasal discharge.   The so-called
"sinus headache" of which many patients complain usually does
not result from sinus disease, as it does not meet the above criteria.

Examination of the ears should be performed carefully to determine the presence of infection or disease.   The patient's hearing
should also be checked.   Posterior fossa tumors will cause a
nerve-type hearing loss of recent onset.   This hearing loss is
also associated with an acoustic neuroma.

Particular attention should be paid to the tongue and palate movements during examination of the mouth.   The possibility of a
tooth abscess should be ruled out.   The pain of temporomandibular joint disease is occasionally caused by a grossly uneven
bite.   This rare pain may be referred to quite distant areas.

Tenderness of the scalp, muscles, or extracranial vessels may
be revealed during palpation of the head and would imply that
the pain arises from extracranial structures, although intracranial causes may also be present.   Temporal arteritis may
present with painful, thickened superficial temporal arteries
with decreased pulsation.   During palpation the bony defects of
the skull resulting from trauma or disease such as fibrous dys-
plasia may be noted.   To rule out temporomandibular joint (TMJ)
disease, the temporomandibular joint should be palpated for
tenderness and crepitations.

Auscultation should be performed over the eyes and the temporal,
occipital, and retroauricular areas of the skull to check for
bruits.   To reduce the amount of blinking and noise interference
while listening over the orbits, the bell of the stethoscope should
be placed gently over one of the patient's closed eyes and then
the patient should open the other eye.   Orbital bruits have been
reported in temporal arteritis and have disappeared following
treatment.   If a bruit is heard, scheduling the patient for angiography should be considered in order to rule out the presence
of a vascular lesion within the skull.   Finally, the carotid arteries in the neck and the supraclavicular areas should also
be auscultated for bruits.

Limitation of motion, spasm, and tenderness should be checked
on the neck.   Tenderness at the neck and trapezius muscles is
often noted in patients with muscle contraction headache and

cervical myalgia. Cervical arthritis, which is a frequent cause
of muscle contraction headaches, may be detected by crepitation.
In some vascular headaches, a prominent factor may be cervical
spondylosis with instability of the cervical spine.

The physical examination should be thorough in order to rule out
any systemic illness which may be associated with the headache
or to determine the presence of any concomitant disease. Headache often accompanies vasculitis or endocarditis, so that a
careful examination of the heart and the cardiovascular system
should be made. In headache with a recent onset, the physician
must be suspicious of an organic cause, and the possibility that
the primary neoplasm is in another part of the body should
be determined.

Neurological Examination

Neurological deficits usually accompany a headache due to intracranial lesions. A systematic examination of the cranial nerves
is indicated in all headache patients. By having the patient identify certain odors (tobacco, oil of peppermint, garlic, etc.) with
each nostril, the first cranial nerve is tested.   An olfactory
groove meningioma may only be identified by anosmia. As discussed previously, the optic nerve is checked by testing the
visual acuity and fields.   Observing the extraocular eye movements will test the third, fourth, and sixth cranial nerves, and
will also rule out ptosis, nystagmus, and pupillary abnormalities.
The symptoms of an aneurysm of the posterior communicating
artery will result in paralysis of the third nerve and include
ptosis, and dilated fixed pupil, and paralysis of upward, downward, and inward gaze.   Paralysis of the lateral gaze is indicative of an aneurysm of the carotid artery adjacent to the sixth
nerve.

The motor function of the muscle groups should be checked after
testing the cranial nerves. Testing of the neck and shoulder
muscles is obtained by having the patient turn the neck against
the resistance of the physician's hand and shrugging the shoulders
against resistance. It is also normal for the physician to be
unable to force the patient's arms downward when the patient is
holding them out horizontally. Attempting to bend the extended
arm and pull down the flexed arm is a test of the biceps and tri-
ceps. The physician should also check the flexion and extension
of the wrist against resistance.

To check the legs for weakness, the physician will try to bend the
extended knee and to straighten the leg flexed at the knee. The feet
are also tested by flexion and extension against the resistance of
the physician's hand.

Testing of the deep tendon reflexes in the limbs is essential. In checking the reflexes, the most important factor to consider is that there should not be a significant difference between tests of each side of the body and on stroking the lateral portion of the plantar surface of the foot (Babinski sign). For example, comparison should be made of the response to plantar stimulation on each side. Extension of the great toe and fanning of the small toes (i. e. , Babinski sign) is indicative of a lesion in the pyramidal system between the motor cortex and the lower spinal cord. The physician should be suspicious of corticospinal tract lesion if there is absence of the abdominal and cremasteric reflexes, especially with hyperactive deep tendon reflexes and particularly if the signs are unilateral. However, in very obese patients or those with surgical scars on the abdomen, the abdominal reflex may be absent.

The neurological examination should include sensory testing. This would involve testing the patient's perception of touch, temperature, position, pinprick, and vibratory sensations. In testing position, the thumb and great toe should be included. Transmission of the position and the vibratory senses are along the same pathways to the thalamus, at which they separate. A lesion above the thalamus should be considered if one those senses is present and the other is absent. To localize areas of neurologic involvement, the corticosensory modalities of object identification, two-point discrimination, and figure writing should be tested.

Observing the patient's gait is very important, to rule out any ataxia or drifting to one side. Limping or lack of arm swinging should be noted. A person with an ataxic gait walks with feet wide apart. Because of leg weakness or foot drop, the person will lift his foot high when walking. The leg is circumducted in patients exhibiting the spastic or scissors gait of corticospinal disease. Gait disturbance associated with headache of recent onset is indicative of a possible organic intracranial lesion. Other tests of coordination include the finger-to-nose and heel-to-shin tests and the Romberg test, with the feet together and the eyes closed. Cerebellar disease is indicated in the patient with inability to perform rapid alternating movements of the hands and feet. The symptoms of cerebellar disease are ipsilateral to a possible lesion.

If any of these basic tests are abnormal, consultation with a neurologist or a neurosurgeon is indicated. There are many more specific and definitive neurologic tests. These ancillary tests include: skull x-rays, echoencephalogram, computerized axial tomography (CAT scan), and radioactive isotope brain scanning.

Unless indicated, invasive studies such as angiography or pneu-
monencephalography should be avoided. The physician may also
consider the use of EEG as a diagnostic tool. It should be remem-
bered that this is not indicated in all headache patients. By per-
forming a thorough physical and neurological examination, the
physician can reassure the headache patient that all attempts to
rule out organic disease have been made.

The motor and sensory divisions of the fifth cranial nerve should
be checked. Because the fifth nerve provides sensation to the
anterior two-thirds of the head and face, it is easily tested. The
fifth and seventh nerve share a function, the corneal reflex, which
is frequently diminished early in patients with acoustic neuroma.
The motor branches of the fifth nerve supplies the pterygoid and
masseter muscles and is tested by palpation as the patient bites down.

Another mixed nerve is the seventh, or facial, nerve. It supplies
the muscles of the face and the sensation of taste to the anterior
two-thirds of the tongue. In the presence of supranuclear or
cortical lesions which cause lower facial muscle paralysis, clos-
ing of the eyes and wrinkling of the forehead may be possible
because of bilateral cortical innervation. Total unilateral facial
paralysis and loss of taste sensation on the anterior two-thirds
of the tongue will be caused by lesions involving the nerve prox-
imal to the junction with the chorda tympani.

Tinnitus and nerve-type deafness will result from an acoustic
neuroma which involves the eighth nerve. In nerve-type deafness,
the patient will note less intense vibration of a tuning fork pressed
against the mastoid process than in one held in front of the ear.

The taste sensation of the posterior one-third of the tongue and
the oropharynx is supplied by the ninth, or glossopharyngeal,
nerve. In lesions involving this nerve, unilateral loss of the
gag reflex is observed. Unilateral vocal cord paralysis and paralysis of the soft palate are presented in lesions of the vagus, or
tenth, nerve. The vagus nerve is also affected by lesions of the
medulla or base of the skull. If weakness in shoulder elevation
or head turning is observed, one must be suspicious of a lesion
involving the eleventh nerve. The hypoglossal, or twelfth, nerve
is checked by observing the tongue for unilateral atrophy, fas-
ciculations, or deviation when protruded.

Chapter 4

Migraine Headache

It is very difficult to define migraine. The best definition is probably Gower's[1]: "Migraine is an affection characterized by paroxysmal nervous disturbance, of which headache is the most constant element. The pain is seldom absent and may exist alone, but is commonly accompanied by nausea and vomiting and is often preceded by some sensory disturbance, especially by some disorder of the sense of sight. The symptoms are frequently one-sided."

The following definitions were agreed to at a meeting of the Research Group on Migraine and Headache[2] (Secretary: Professor Arnold Friedman) of the World Federation of Neurology (President: Doctor Macdonald Critchley) at its meeting in London, April 22, 1969.

Migraine: "A familial disorder characterized by recurrent attacks of headache widely variable in intensity, frequency, and duration. Attacks are commonly unilateral and are usually associated with anorexia, nausea, and vomiting. In some cases they are preceded by, or associated with, neurological and mood disturbances. All of the above characteristics are not necessarily present in each attack."

A. Conditions generally accepted as falling within the above definition.

    1. Classical migraine, in which headache is preceded or accompanied by transient focal neurological phenomena — for example, visual, sensory, or speech disturbances.

    2. Nonclassical migraine, which is not associated with sharply defined focal neurological disturbances. This is the more common variety encountered.

B.   Conditions which may fall within the category of migraine.

    1.   <u>Cluster headaches.</u> Unilateral intense pain involving
the eye and head on one side usually associated with
flushing, nasal congestion, and lacrimation, attacks
recurring one or more times daily and lasting for 20 to
120 minutes. Such bouts commonly continue for weeks
or months and are separated by remissions of months
or years (synonyms: Harris's ciliary or migrainous
neuralgia, Horton's histaminic cephalalgia.)

    2.   <u>Facial "migraine. "</u> Unilateral episodic facial pain as-
sociated with symptoms suggestive either of migraine
or cluster headache (synonym: "lower-half" headache).

    3.   <u>Ophthalmoplegic "migraine. "</u> Episodic migrainelike
attacks associated with objective evidence of paresis
of the extraocular muscles, usually those supplied by
the third nerve, often outlasting the headache. A structural abnormality must be excluded before this diagnosis
is made.

    4.   <u>Hemiplegic "migraine. "</u> A rare condition, which may
exhibit a dominant inheritance, characterized by episodic migrainous attacks associated with hemiplegia
and outlasting the headache.

<u>Pathogenesis</u>

Migraine is thought to be a reaction pattern to a number of factors
caused by an interaction between inherited traits and exogenous
or endogenous factors.   The inherited traits consist of two abnormalities: (1) neurovascular instability and (2) platelet changes.

Different exogenous and endogenous factors can trigger the sudden release of serotonin from the dense bodies of the platelets.
Serotonin produces capillaric dilatation and constriction of the
extracranial and some intracranial arteries. The constrictor
effect is the cause of the aura that precedes the headache in 10%
to 20% of migraines. Serotonin is absorbed by the blood vessels
and nearby tissues where it works together with kinin to produce
inflammation. Serotonin is metabolized in the tissues, and this
accounts for a rapid drop in blood serotonin during migraine
attacks. The drop causes a rebound effect with vasodilation of
both arteries and constriction of the capillary vessels. Both
arterial distension and inflammation give rise to headache.

A number of trigger factors are going to affect migraine: stress, hormones, and diet with foods containing tryamine, monosodium glutamate, nitrites, and nitrates. Ergotamine, when taken in excess, can cause rebound headaches. Estrogen, when given to menopausal women or used as a contraceptive, can precipitate migraine.

The frequency and severity of migraine may be increased by a number of conditions: depression, high altitude, moderate or severe hypertension, and collagen disorders. It should be stressed that although allergy has been considered by some authors to be a precipitant of migraine, most headache specialists do not consider migraine an allergic condition. Also, there is no relationship between epilepsy and migraine.

Clinical Manifestations

Migraine headaches are intermittent, usually unilateral headaches that are frequently associated with irritability, nausea, photophobia, vomiting, and diarrhea. The pain may be limited to half of the head at the onset, and it might radiate to the opposite side later in the course of the headache. The body participates in migraine, and very frequently the patient complains of vertigo, tremors, pallor, excessive perspiration, and chills. The patient may have an aura a few minutes prior to the migraine attack. The aura may consist of scotoma, hemianopsia, paresthesias, or hemiparesis. During the headache attack, the patient appears sick. His face is pale and the skin is sweaty. The blood vessels on the side of the pain may be dilated and tender; the skin of the skull ipsilateral to the pain is sore. The patient appears tense and irritable. He speaks in a very low voice as if he is trying to avoid increasing the pain and very often seems confused. The patient may become irritable, compulsive, and hostile, and his memory and concentration are very poor.

The frequency of migraine varies from 1-3 times per week to 1 every 2 years, and the duration ranges between several hours and several days. The intensity may be moderate, severe, or incapacitating pain.

Abortive Treatment

When migraine is very mild, the use of aspirin or acetaminophen may be sufficient to abort the attack (see flowchart of p. 33). However, migraine headaches are usually of moderate to severe intensity and rarely respond to such mild medications.

The drug of choice in the treatment of acute migraine attacks is ergotamine tartrate. Ergotamine tartrate is a vasoconstrictor that is mainly metabolized in the liver. Its elimination half-life is about 6.5 hr, but some metabolites are excreted for 35 hr. It has many side effects such as abdominal cramps, epigastric discomfort, diarrhea, nausea, vomiting, painful uterine contractions, and intermittent claudication or acute arterial occlusion. Mild side effects such as nausea and vomiting are found in about 35% of the patients, and the more severe toxic effects in about 1 in every 600 patients. Ergotamine may be given orally, sublingually, by inhalation, rectally, or parenterally. The oral and sublingual dosages are 2 mg at the onset of the attack and 1 mg every half-hour, not to exceed 6 mg/day or 10 mg/week. By inhalation, one dose can be taken every 4 min up to a maximum of 6 doses/day. Rectally, a suppository of 2 mg can be taken and repeated 1 hr later if needed. A maximum of 4 mg/day and 10 mg/week is allowed. The recommended dosage for intramuscular or subcutaneous routes is 0.25 to 0.5 mg, and the maximum dosage allowed is 1 mg/week. The effectiveness of ergotamine is related to the speed at which it is administered and the route used. Ergotamine's effectiveness is also dependent on how early it is taken in an acute attack. Several reports have been made on the various routes of administration. However, definitive studies have differed within individual preference and idiosyncrasy.

There are several contraindications for the use of ergotamine: pregnancy, coronary heart disease, peripheral vascular disease, significant hepatic or renal dysfunction, thyrotoxicosis, severe hypertension, sepsis, anemia, Raynaud's phenomenon, and thrombophlebitis.

Dihydroergotamine is another medication with actions, metabolism, side effects, and indications similar to those of ergotamine tartrate. It can only be given by intramuscular route, and the usual dosage is 1 mg at the onset of the migraine attack and repeated every hour to a maximum of 3 mg/day.

When ergotamine is taken frequently, it increases the frequency of migraine because it causes rebound headaches. To avoid these headaches, ergotamine should never be given two days in a row. It is advisable not to administer ergotamine in those patients who have more than two migraine headaches per week. In these patients the use of the combination of a mild vasoconstrictor such as isometheptene and an antiemetic agent may be used. Isometheptene is contraindicated in patients with hypertension, heart disease, and peripheral vascular disease.

Occasionally patients will have prolonged migraine attacks. It is thought that a sterile inflammation has occurred around the vessels participating in the migraine headache. The headaches may last 2 to 7 days in these cases. These patients benefit from the use of steroids. Dexamethasone 16 mg intramuscularly can be given if the headache does not disappear in the first 24 hours. It usually has dramatic results.

Prophylactic Treament

Various types of drugs, including antihypertensive, antiserotonin agents, antidepressants, and platelet antagonists, have been found effective in migraine (see flowchart on p. 33).

Propranolol

Propranolol has been proven to be a useful agent in the prophylactic treatment of migraine. Propranolol has numerous mechanisms of action which may contribute to its effectiveness in migraine. The action of the drug includes the following: (1) it blocks beta receptors and therefore can prevent arterial dilation; (2) it blocks catecholamine-induced platelet aggregation; (3) it decreases platelet adhesiveness; (4) it prevents elevation of coagulation factors during epinephrine release; (5) it shifts the hemoglobin-oxygen dissociation curve, promoting release of oxygen to tissues; (6) it inhibits renin secretion; and (7) it blocks catecholamine-induced lipolysis. The blocking of lipolysis produces a decrease in arachidonic acid, a precursor of prostaglandins, and consequently results in a decrease in prostaglandins. The decrease in prostaglandins accounts for the inhibition of platelet aggregation.

In carefully selected patients, propranolol is the drug of choice for prophylaxis of migraine. Patients should not have asthma, chronic obstructive lung disease, congestive heart failure, or atrioventricular conduction disturbances. Propranolol should not be given to patients who are being treated with insulin, oral hypoglycemic agents, or monoamine oxidase (MAO) inhibitors. The drug is especially helpful for migraineurs with severe hypertension, angina pectoris, or thyrotoxicosis, in whom ergot preparations are contraindicated. In such situations, one medication relieves the headache as well as the coexisting disorder.

Propranolol is taken orally in a dosage of 20 to 40 mg q. i. d. In most patients, we start with 20 mg q. i. d. for a week and then increase the fourth, or bedtime dose to 40 mg. The plasma half-life of propranolol is 3 hours. However, its beta-blocking action seems to last about 12 hr. Therefore, twice-daily

administration may also be effective.   Propranolol should not
be withdrawn suddenly in patients with coronary heart disease
because this might exacerbate coronary ischemia and lead to
unstable angina or myocardial infarction.

As previously mentioned, propranolol is not suitable for patients
taking insulin or oral hypoglycemic drugs.   Hypoglycemia produces liberation of epinephrine, with resulting tachycardia and
palpitations.   Propranolol blocks these compensatory and warning mechanisms.   Furthermore, since propranolol blocks beta
receptors in blood vessels, alpha receptors predominate and the
liberated epinephrine may cause severe hypertension.

Methysergide

Because of its many side effects, methysergide is only considered as a treatment when other prophylactic agents have failed.
Methysergide is believed to be effective since it blocks the inflammatory and vasoconstrictor effects of serotonin.   The drug
is excreted in the urine and has an eliminating half-life of 2. 7
hr, although some metabolites are excreted for about 10 hr.

Its vasoconstrictor effects are rarely noted except in patients
with a tendency to develop ischemic complications. These complications will only occur in about 2% of the patients. In patients
who have taken methysergide for a prolonged period, methysergide can produce fibrotic syndromes, such as endocardial or
retroperitoneal fibrosis.   Intravenous pyelograms should be
ordered every 6 months in order to avoid these complications.
Every 6 months, the patient should be advised to discontinue the
drug for at least 1 month.   Other side effects may prevent the
use of this medication in about one-third of the patients.   These
include: gastrointestinal pain, nausea, vomiting, diarrhea, dizziness, anxiety, drowsiness, hallucinations, and, on occasion,
psychotic reactions.   Other symptoms which have been noted
include: weight gain, hair loss, and muscle cramps.

The usual dose of methysergide is 4 to 8 mg/day. It is effective
in about 60% of migraine sufferers. This drug is contraindicated
in patients with peptic ulcer, pregnancy, thrombophlebitis, or
peripheral vascular or coronary heart disease.

Clonidine

This antihypertensive drug has also been recommended for prophylaxis of migraine, but consensus has not been reached con-
cerning its effectiveness.

Some investigators consider clonidine the drug of choice for patients who are sensitive to foods containing tyramine. Such patients constitute about 30% of the migraine population. Other studies could not demonstrate any significant effects of clonidine. We have found clonidine to be useful in some patients with migraine but, in general, to be much less effective than propranolol.

Clonidine acts centrally by inhibiting sympathetic outflow from the vasomotor center in the medulla and peripherally by reducing the response of blood vessels to both vasoconstrictor and vasodilator substances.

The drug is given orally, beginning in a dosage of 0.1 mg b.i.d. and slowly increasing to a maximum of 2.4 mg daily. This drug should not be discontinued abruptly because of the danger of causing severe hypertensive crisis. Such hypertensive crises are due to a marked increase in secretion of catecholamines from the adrenal medulla and may be fatal. If clonidine has to be discontinued, the dosage should be reduced gradually over 2 to 4 days.

Side effects with clonidine are frequent but mild. Patients may complain of drowsiness, dryness of mouth, constipation, and occasional disturbance of ejaculation. Mild orthostatic hypotension occurs in 50% of patients. Depression may develop, but tricyclic antidepressants should not be used because they inhibit clonidine's activity. Retinal degeneration has occurred with clonidine use, making periodic retinal examinations necessary.

Antiserotonin Agents

The stress during the past decade on serotonin's role in the pathogenesis of migraine has led to the introduction of new antiserotonin drugs for migraine therapy. The first one, pizotifen, is widely used in Europe but has not been used in the United States. This drug has an antiamine effect against serotonin and histamine as well as against acetylcholine, tryptamine, and catecholamines. It is usually given in a dosage of 0.5 mg t.i.d. After an oral dose of 1 mg, maximum serum concentration is reached in 5 to 7 hr, with minimal activity after 12 hr. Pizotifen is excreted mainly by the kidneys and has a biologic half-life of 26 hr.

The efficacy of pizotifen has been confirmed in several short-term and long-term clinical studies, with success rates ranging from 40% to 68%. The main side effects are weight gain, drowsiness, and dizziness.

Bromocriptine

This ergot medication is being evaluated for efficacy in migraine.
It is a semisynthetic ergot alkaloid free of cardiovascular and
oxytocic actions.   Bromocriptine suppresses prolactin secretion and has been used successfully for treatment of the premenstrual syndrome.

Investigators have observed that migraine was likely to occur
when prolactin secretion is elevated — for example, with stress,
oversleeping, premenstrual period, or estrogen or oral contraceptive therapy.   Research studies have tested bromocriptine in seven women with menstrual migraine and found that in
10 to 12 menstrual cycles the women were completely free of
migraine.   The drug was initially given at a dosage of 2. 5 mg
with the evening meal.   The dosage was increased at 4-day in-
tervals to 2. 5 mg b. i. d. and then to 2. 5 g t. i. d.   Among the
side effects were nausea, dizziness and lightheadedness, leg
cramps, gastric discomfort, diarrhea, flatulence, and constipation.

We believe that headaches which occur only during the premenstrual or menstrual period should not be treated with continuous
daily drug therapy.   Therefore, on several occasions we have
tried bromocriptine[3] during the premenstrual and menstrual
period only, but without success.

Antidepressants

In the past decade, this class of drugs has also been tried in
migraine.   Some investigators have reported on the effect of
the MAO-inhibitor phenelzine. These investigators concluded
that MAO inhibitors are worthy of trial in patients who have not
responded to other therapies. However, there are potential serious side effects with these medications. We reserve phenelzine,
45 mg/day, for previously unresponsive patients.

In the late 1960s, amitryptiline was occasionally mentioned for
prophylaxis of migraine. [4] The beneficial effects of amitryptiline in migraine were reported in the 1970s. The improvement was
not related to the drug's antidepressant action, suggesting that
other mechanisms of action might be responsible for controlling
the headaches.

Amitriptyline can block reuptake of catecholamines and serotonin
at nerve endings in both central and peripheral nervous systems;
has anticholinergic, antihistaminic, and antiserotonergic effects;
and may interfere with release of norephinephrine at nerve endings.

A double-blind multicenter combined study was subsequently undertaken to determine whether amitriptyline was more effective than placebo in reducing the frequency and severity of migraine headaches. Results showed amitriptyline to be no more effective than placebo.

We feel that amitriptyline is extremely helpful in mixed migraine and muscle contraction headaches. In many such cases, depression is a significant component of the disorder.

Platelet Antagonists

During the past few years, a strong relationship has been established between platelet changes and migraine which has given rise to the use of platelet antagonists in prevention of migraine attacks. Among the important changes known to occur in the platelets of patients with migraine are: (1) increased aggregability to serotonin due to greater capacity of the platelet membraine for uptake of serotonin; (2) chronic hyperaggregability in response to other substances; and (3) a decrease of MAO type B.

Release of serotonin from platelets initiates a migraine attack and may account for the sterile inflammation that is so important for development of the headache. In addition, an increase in platelet adhesiveness occurs during the headache phase of migraine that parallels the increase in platelet serotonin during the headache aura.

The three major platelet antagonists are aspirin, sulfinpyrazone, and dipyridamole. Aspirin inhibits cyclooxygenase, an enzyme which transforms arachidonic acid to prostaglandin E, which in turn changes to thromboxane. Thromboxane causes platelet aggregation. Aspirin also destroys the thrombosthenin of platelets.

Like aspirin, sulfinpyrazone inactivates cyclooxygenase. Dipyridamole works in a different way, inhibiting phosphodiesterase and thus increasing cyclic adenosine monophosphate (cAMP). The cAMP inhibits release of adenosine diphosphate (ADP), the substance which initiates the chain of events leading to platelet aggregation.

Therapeutic dosage of aspirin has shown it to be of some benefit in the prevention of migraine: 9 to 12 migraineurs improved with aspirin therapy. Further studies are needed to assess the value of platelet antagonists in the prevention of migraine.

TREATING MIGRAINE

(Decision points in heavy outline)

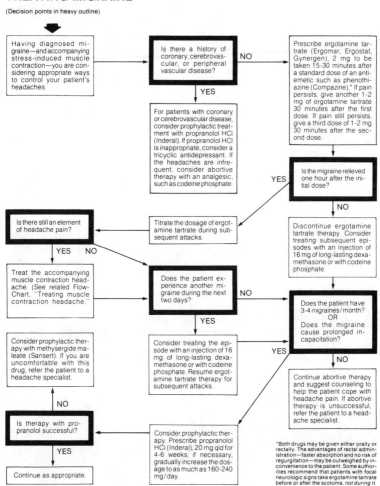

Chapter 5

Cluster Headache

Cluster headache has been known under many pseudonyms: migrainous neuralgia, histamine headache, Horton's histamine cephalalgia, erythromelalgia of the head, ciliary neuralgia, and greater superficial pertrosal neuralgia. It has also been known as Raeder's syndrome or Sluder's syndrome, but some consider these as separate syndromes, although this has not been documented. However, in the 1950s, a common term, "cluster headache," was selected as an appropriate name for this condition.

It is characterized by severe pain behind or around one eye which spreads on the affected side. Conjunctival injection, tearing, nasal congestion, rhinorrhea, sweating and flushing on the portion of the face where the headache is prominent, and partial Horner's syndrome are quite often associated with the pain.

In the majority of patients, cluster headache strikes in the second or third decade. Attacks occur mainly in the spring and fall and are brief, lasting anywhere from several minutes to several hours, but rarely more than 4 hours. They occur once or many times per day, appearing most often during the night, and continue over a period of weeks or months. The headaches may then disappear for six months or for a year or two, only to return at a later time. In some unfortunate patients, an attack may be continuous for years.

The pain of cluster headache is usually described as throbbing or pulsating. Many patients describe it as severe and constant. Others liken it to a knife cutting into their head. The pain is of such magnitude and severity that patients have attempted or committed suicide during a series of attacks.

The dietary factor best known to trigger an attack during a cluster series is ingestion of an alcoholic beverage. An injection of histamine or the administration of nitroglycerin can also trigger a cluster headache.

Comparison of Cluster and Migraine Headaches

Most headache experts believe that cluster and migraine headaches are of vascular origin, but they still do not agree whether to consider cluster headache a variant of migraine or an entirely different disorder. Those who link these diseases stress the similarities, while those who distinguish them stress the differences. Table 5-1 contrasts the features of cluster and migraine headache and may be helpful in differentiating the diagnosis.

Table 5-1. Contrasting Features of Cluster and Migraine Headaches

Feature	Cluster	Migraine
Location of pain	Always unilateral, periorbital	Unilateral, occasionally bilateral
Age at onset	20-50 years	10-40 years
Sex incidence	99% male	65-75% female
Occurrence of attacks	Daily for several weeks to several months	Intermittent, 2-8 times per month
Seasonal occurrence	More common in spring and fall	No variance
Number of attacks	1 to 6 per day	1 to 8 per month
Duration of pain	10 min to 3 hr	4 to 48 hr
Prodromes	Absent	25-30% of cases
Nausea and vomiting	2-5%	86%
Blurring of vision	Infrequent	Frequent
Lacrimation	Frequent	Infrequent
Nasal congestion	70%	Uncommon
Ptosis	30%	1-2%
Polyuria	2%	40%
Family History of vascular headaches	7%	90%
Miosis	50%	Absent
Chemical Changes		
Decrease in plasma serotonin	None	80%
Rise in plasma histamine	90%	None
Rise in CSF acetylcholine	30%	None

Chronic Paroxysmal Hemicrania

The headaches of chronic paroxysmal hemicrania (CPH) are considered atypical cluster headaches because of their high daily
frequency and brief duration. The location of these headaches
may be in atypical areas and can be provoked by movements. Indomethacin is the treatment of choice in this syndrome. Also
observed in CPH are multiple jabs and background vascular headaches. This syndrome is characterized by their periods of 15
or more attacks per day, unilaterality of the pain, and the complete response to indomethacin.

Cluster Headache Variant

This syndrome has recently been identified. It too is characterized by atypical cluster headaches, multiple jabs, and background vascular headaches. The headaches occur several times
per day, and in contrast to chronic paroxysmal hemicrania the
affected patients usually do not have any headache-free periods.
They differ from typical cluster headaches in their duration, frequency, location, and frequent shifting. Multiple jabs are sharp
pains of variable severity and location and are short-lasting. The
final characteristic, background vascular headache is continuous,
chronic, often unilateral, of variable severity, and may begin to
throb during exertion or throbs at rest. In a recent study, 83%
of the patients reviewed had a good response to indomethacin.
The response to indomethacin was variable in comparison to CPH.

Treatment of Cluster Headache

Once cluster headache has been diagnosed and the differentia-
tion from other conditions is clearly established, treatment in
most instances is not difficult (see flowchart on pp. 38-39).
Initally, during a series of attacks, certain habits (consumption
of alcoholic beverages and smoking) should be discouraged in
order to prevent symptoms from recurring.

Abortive Therapy

Ergotamine tartrate may be used to abort a mild attack. The
route of administration can be varied to suit the patient's needs.
The drug may be given orally in tablet form (Cafergot, Gynergen,
Migral, Wigraine), rectally in the form of suppositories (Cafergot, Wigraine), sublingually (Ergomar, Ergostat) or by inhalation (Medihaler).

In patients with severe attacks, it may be necessary to teach them to administer ergotamine tartrate parenterally. For this purpose, the use of dihydroergotamine (DHE-45) given parenternally at 1 cc is recommended. When ergotamine tartrate is contraindicated because of poor circulation, cardiac disease, cerebrovascular disease, or altered peripheral circulation, the patients may be given isometheptene mucate (Midrin). An individual attack which does not respond to ergotamine tartrate can be aborted by administering oxygen at 8 to 10 L/min for 10 min by oxygen mask. However, this treatment may be effective in only a small proportion of patients.

Prophylactic Therapy

Patients whose headaches are so severe that they cannot be controlled by abortive methods may respond to prophylaxis. Ergotamine tartrate, 3 to 5 mg, may be administered orally to prevent attacks. Since many of the attacks occur at night, a larger dose (sometimes 2 to 3 mg) may be given at bedtime and a smaller dose during the day. Patients who do not respond to ergotamine tartrate prophylaxis may be given 6 to 12 mg of methysergide (Sansert) in 2 mg tablets, depending on the severity of the attacks.

Steroids may be used in some instances where patients are not responsive to ergotamine tartrate or methysergide. Excellent results have been observed in using prednisone, usually 40 mg/day. If this dosage is insufficient, it may be necessary to give a steroid in combination with either ergotamine tartrate or methysergide.

None of the aforementioned drugs can be taken for a prolonged period without risking potentially hazardous side effects. However, they can be safely administered for the limited duration of most cluster attacks.

About 5% of cluster headaches are chronic, occurring throughout the year. Recently, Ekbom of Sweden has shown that many patients with chronic cluster headache can be helped by the use of lithium carbonate 300 mg t.i.d.[5]. Of course, the blood level of lithium should be checked every 4 to 6 weeks and kept between 0.5 to 1.5 mEq/L.

TREATING CLUSTER HEADACHE

(Decision points in heavy outline)

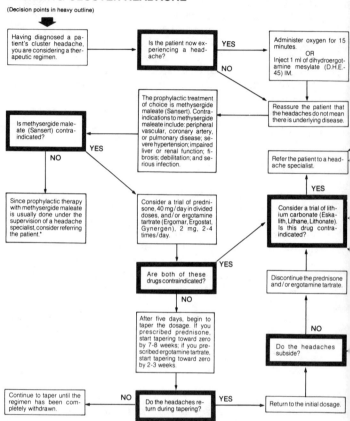

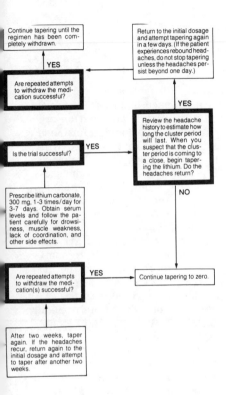

Continue tapering until the regimen has been completely withdrawn.

YES

Are repeated attempts to withdraw the medication successful?

Return to the initial dosage and attempt tapering again in a few days. (If the patient experiences rebound headaches, do not stop tapering unless the headaches persist beyond one day.)

YES

Is the trial successful?

YES

Review the headache history to estimate how long the cluster period will last. When you suspect that the cluster period is coming to a close, begin tapering the lithium. Do the headaches return?

NO

Prescribe lithium carbonate, 300 mg, 1-3 times/day for 3-7 days. Obtain serum levels and follow the patient carefully for drowsiness, muscle weakness, lack of coordination, and other side effects.

Are repeated attempts to withdraw the medication(s) successful?

YES

Continue tapering to zero.

After two weeks, taper again. If the headaches recur, return again to the initial dosage and attempt to taper after another two weeks.

*Some authorities prescribe a combination of methysergide maleate and a corticosteroid. If you decide to manage the patient yourself, examine the heart, lungs, urine, and circulatory system monthly. Interrupt drug therapy for 3-4 weeks every 3-4 months for IVP and other appropriate tests.

Chapter 6

Muscle Contraction Headache

Eighty percent of the headache patients seen by either the family
physician or the generalist suffer from muscle contraction or
tension headaches. It manifests itself in relationship to stress,
depression, emotional conflicts, fatigue, or repressed hostility.
These problems may not be evident to the sufferer. The physiological response which follows is a reflex dilatation of the external cranial vessels and a contraction of the skeletal muscles
of the head, neck, or face, resulting in the characteristic pain
of muscle contraction headache.

Muscle contraction headaches can occur at any age but are more
common in adulthood when the frustrations of life tend to domi-
nate. A classic review by one of the authors found that the majority of his patients were female and that about 40% had a family
history of headache, compared to 70% of migraine sufferers with
a family history of headache. The onset of most of his patients'
headaches was between the ages of 20 and 40. Thirty percent
had daily pain, and 20% had persistent complaints.

The amount of muscle tone at the head and scalp are determined
by the degree of activity of a special group of anterial horn cells
called the fusimotor or gamma efferent neurons. A small in-
hibitory nerve cell called the Renshaw cell acts on the alpha
motor neurons supplying the extrafusal fibers. The corticol,
afferent, and efferent pathways are also directly related to
these symptoms, and it is the interreaction between these symptoms that maintains the state of muscle tone. Therefore, we
feel that various cortical functions or limbic functions may ad-
versely influence this maintenance system, causing it to produce
excessive muscle contraction which can then lead to pain. It may
be maintained by itself, more or less, as in "the dog chasing
its own tail" principle. The excessive muscle contraction producing the pain leads to anxiety and reinforces the excessive
muscle contraction, thereby starting a vicious and self-
sustaining circle.

Muscle contraction headache may occur as a secondary phenomenon when there is head or face pain from other causes. Examples are headache associated with sustained muscle contraction due to faulty posture, cervical spondylosis, discogenic disease,
bony anomalies of the occipital-cervical junction, cervical cord
and posterior cranial fossa tumors, and disorders of the tempo-
mandibular joint.

The tension headache is a steady, nonpulsatile ache. Additional
descriptive terms include: "tightness" bitemporally or at the
occiput; "bandlike" sensations about the head, which may become
caplike in distribution; "viselike" ache; "weight, " "pressure, "
"drawing, " and "soreness. " Distinct cramplike sensations and
a "feeling as if the neck and upper back were in a cast" are other
terms used to describe the pain.

These head pains and other sensations occur frequently in the
forehead and temples or in the back of the head and neck, as
well as at other sites.   They may be unilateral or bilateral, involving the temporal, occipital, parietal, or frontal regions, or
any combination of these sites.   Frequently, there is a soreness
on combing or brushing the hair or when putting on a hat.   Although muscle contraction headache may be fleeting, with frequent changes in the site and intensity, this is the type of headache which, localized in one region, may be sustained with varying
intensity for weeks, months, or even years.   The intensity of
the headache may be diminished by assuming certain individually
favored positions.   The patient may limit the motion of the head,
neck, and jaws because it decreases his discomfort.   There may
be less discomfort when the head is supported with the hands.

Within the diffusely aching muscle tissues of the head, neck,
and upper back, there may be found on palpation one or more
tender areas, or nodules, which are sharply localized. Pressure
on contracted, tender muscles may augment headache intensity
and may elicit tinnitus, vertigo, and lacrimation. These features
may also occur spontaneously.   Such pressure on tender areas
causes radiation of the pain to adjacent portions of the head.
Muscle contraction headache may also be aggravated by shiver-
ing from exposure to cold.

Diagnosis of Muscle Contraction Headache

The diagnosis of muscle contraction headache is made through
a thorough and careful headache history accompanied with a
complete neurological examination to rule out organic etiology.
A careful survey of emotional factors is essential in forming the

diagnosis of mucle contraction headache. Inquiring if the patient has chronic feelings of tension, nervousness, irritability, or difficulty relaxing is important. It should also be determined if the patient has symptoms of anxiety such as shaking of the hands, a lump in the throat, rapid heartbeat, or tightness in the chest or lower abdomen.

Since headache often accompanies depression, a careful inventory of depressive symptoms is important. The depressed patient may exhibit many physicial symptoms, with headache being the primary one. Sleep disturbance in the form of early and frequent awakening is very prominent. The patient may have other physical complaints, such as shortness of breath, constipation, weight loss, feelings of fatigue, decreased sexual drive, palpitations, and menstrual changes.

The patient may also exhibit emotional complaints and look "blue," in low spirits, or sad as you interview them. Some of these patients will cry spontaneously as you talk to them. They will express feelings of guilt, hopelessness, unworthiness, and unreality, and may have some anxiety along with their depression. There may be a basic fear of insanity, physical disease or death, and these patients will ruminate over the past, present, and future. Psychic complaints may present, such as poor concentration, loss of interest, ambition, indecisiveness, poor memory, and suicidal thoughts. These patients view morning as the worst time of the day and may have a diurnal variation to their pain. It is important in elderly patients to determine if they are depressed, as many of these patients have been diagnosed as senile when a depression is actually present.

Chronic muscle contraction headache is constant and unremitting. It may be present for weeks, months, years, or decades. The pain may affect the same areas of the head as the acute type and is characteristically bilateral. Some patients describe a tightband, like a tight skull cap, or hatband distribution to the headache.

There are two types of muscle contraction headache: episodic and chronic. The episodic type is quite common, and many of these patients never seek the help of a physician since their headaches are relieved by various over-the-counter analgesics. A problem starts when the analgesics are taken on a daily basis or in excessive amounts. The characteristics of the episodic muscle contraction headache are mild to moderate pain involving the temporal, frontal, vertex or occipital, and cervical regions

separately or in any combination. The headaches are usually
described as occurring bilaterally and may be triggered by such
factors as fatigue, acute family crisis, and stressful workloads.

Treatment of Muscle Contraction Headache

If the headache is occurring on an intermittent basis, the treatment of the muscle contraction headache includes common analgesics and sedatives (see flowchart on p. 45). Sometimes many
of these patients will have a basic fear that they have an underlying fatal disorder such as a brain tumor or an aneurysm. A
thorough history and a neurological examination may be all the
reassurance a patient requires. If there are psychological problems, an inventory should be made of their psychogenic deter-
minents such as marital relationships, occupations, social relationships, life stresses, personality traits, habits, methods
of handling tension situations, or sexual problems. The physician
should be detailed in the inventory. Sometimes discussing problems with the patient will be sufficient. Some patients will require
psychotherapy, and should be referred for a significant problem.
A few patients may be helped with heat and massage, applied
locally, but the response is usually minimal.

The tricyclic antidepressants are probably the most useful of all
therapeutic agents. These compounds interfere with the uptake
of the neurotransfer amines into the synaptic stores, resulting
in the increased availability of epinephrine and norepinephrine
and other such amines which may promote their pharmacological
activity. If anxiety is a primary factor, the addition of a mild
tranquilizer with the tricyclic antidepressant may be indicated.
The use of amitriptyline or doxepin in large nighttime doses is
helpful because these individuals will have a sleep disturbance.
For the patient who is obviously depressed but does not report
a sleep disturbance, nortriptyline or protriptyline on a daily
basis is indicated. Propranolol is sometimes helpful and can
be used in combination with the tricyclic compounds. It has been
shown to have an anxiolytic effect, which may explain its beneficial response. If the patients presents with a mixed headache
syndrome — vascular headache with tension headache — propranolol
may be especially beneficial in these cases. If the mixed-headache
patient is unresponsive to any of these forms of therapy, the
use of the monoamine oxidase (MAO) inhibitors may be indicated,
primarily phenelzine (Nardil) 15 mg, t. i. d. It is well to remem-
ber that this patient needs a special diet, and an irresponsible
patient should not be started on an MAO inhibitor.

Biofeedback can be of great value in the patient with muscle contraction headache who is not depressed. It is important to use biofeedback in intelligent patients and in patients who are not adverse to participating in a method to train physiological functions. The purpose of biofeedback in the treatment of muscle contraction headache is to train the patients to use their thought process through electromyographic relaxation techniques in order to override the physiological disturbance that occurs with this disorder. With good instruction and adequate practice, the biofeedback process, in itself, may become more or less automatic, thus becoming effective.

TREATING MUSCLE CONTRACTION HEADACHE

(Decision points in heavy outline)

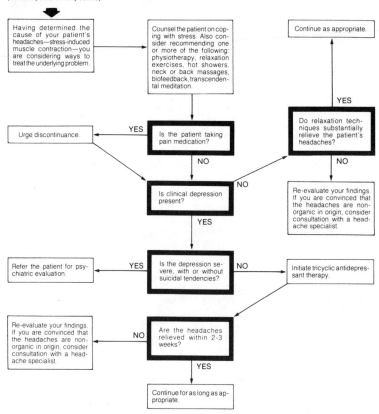

Chapter 7

Organic Causes of Headache Associated With Primary Disease
of the Nervous System

Anyone seeking medical attention for headache should be carefully evaluated for clues that might indicate possible intracranial
or systemic disease.

It is obvious that different possibilities are raised by a patient
who presents himself for the first time in his life with severe
headache and another one who has had recurrent headache for
over a period of years.

In most instances, the diagnosis of headaches associated with
intracranial or systemic disease is made primarily on the basis
of associated physical and laboratory findings; however, an important first step in establishing a diagnosis and management
program is to take a comprehensive history, including a medical
and family history and a review of the psychological and social
background of the patient.

Headache resulting from intracranial lesions has the following
pattern. The headache is usually a steady, nonthrobbing, deep,
dull ache, which may awaken the patient from a sound sleep. It
is often intermittent but continuous in a small number of patients.
Although sometimes severe, it is rarely as intense as the headaches of migraine or certain febrile illnesses unless it is due to
a ruptured aneurysm or meningitis. Coughing, straining at
stool, or changing in posture, such as bending forward, may
produce or aggravate the headache. In the presence of increased
intracranial pressure vomiting may occur, at times without pre-
ceding nausea. The unilateral pain usually occurs on the same
side as the tumor, but the pain becomes generalized in the presence of increased intracranial pressure.

Pleocytosis and an increase in spinal fluid protein are rarely
encountered in the early phase of any of these conditions, but an
increase in spinal fluid protein is a common sequellum of subarachnoid hemorrhage and longitudinal sinus thrombosis.

Early-stage meningitis may be easily mistaken for grippelike illness—even the onset of neck stiffness attributes to myalgia.

Postlumbar Puncture Headache

Headache is a very common phenomenon following lumbar puncture. An average incidence of 36% after diagnostic lumbar puncture has been reported.

Headaches may begin within 6 to 48 hr after lumbar puncture. The effect of body posture or position on the headache is striking, in that the headache is most severe when the patient is upright, and relieved or diminished when the patient is supine. Headache may be frontal, occipital, diffuse. It commonly lasts 24 to 48 hr, but in some patients it may persist for weeks.

The probable mechanism is leakage of cerebrospinal fluid through the dural-arachnoidal puncture, producing dilatation and traction of intracranial vessels.

Cough (Exertional) Headache

In the large majority of patients with transient pain headache precipitated by coughing, sneezing, and so on— there are no serious inferences; the condition is self-limited. However, 10% of such individuals harbor intracranial lesions, usually located in the posterior fossa.

Arnold-Chiari malformation and basilar impression are the most common abnormalities found. Otherwise, subdural hematoma, hemispheric, brain stem, and cerebellar tumors, and other posterior fossa tumors also may be responsible.

Following treatment, 30% of patients remain symptom-free for 5 years; the other 70% are improved and remain headache-free for 10 years. All such patients should undergo computerized axial tomography (CAT scan) exam annually.

Many patients with benign exertional headaches respond to Indomethacin, 75 mg daily.

Cranial Inflammation

Headache with fever should always first bring to mind the possibility of meningitis. It rarely presents so acutely as to resemble subarachnoid hemorrhage. Many agents can cause inflammation of the meninges, including blood, viral, fungal, or bacterial infection and even metastatic disease to the meninges, such as lymphoma. The symptoms are determined by the type of structure involved, the degree of inflammation, and the location of the inflammatory process. Meningitis headache is frequently holocranial, but tends to be worse occipitally. This may be due to the extreme reflex spasm of the cervical musculature. Meningitis in its earliest state with mild to moderate headache and minimal stiffness of the neck may be mistaken for grippe-like or flu illness. In aseptic meningitis, the clinical manifestations include a more severe headache than is usually associated with simple febrile states. Virus infections are the principal causes of aseptic meningitis; however, a similar cerebrospinal fluid reaction may also characterize parameningeal inflammation, such as brain abscess, encephalitis, epidural or subdural abscess, and otitis media, retropharyngeal abscess, and superior longitudinal sinus thrombosis.

In patients suspect of meningitis, the major diagnostic procedure is lumbar puncture. The examiner should be aware of any recent use of antibiotics by the patient, since these may significantly modify the spinal fluid values from those seen in bacterial meningitis to those usually found in viral meningitis.

Four major conditions, which have in common a complaint of severe headache and/or the presence of resistance to anterior flexion of the neck, may be mistaken for meningitis:

1. Retropharyngeal abscess, particularly in children

2. Superior longitudinal sinus thrombosis

3. Subarachnoid hemorrhage

4. Meningismus that may accompany certain infections such as typhoid fever

Subarachnoid Hemorrhage

Bleeding into the subarachnoid space may take place after head trauma, which is the most common cause of intracranial hemorrhage or may be secondary to intracerebral hemorrhage or occur spontaneously by bleeding from preexisting aneurysms or vascular malformations. Less commonly, bleeding may be a manifestation of a blood dyscrasia, hemorrhage from intracranial tumor, or some form of arteritis. The clinical presentation for all spontaneous subarachnoid hemorrhage is the acute onset of a severe headache. The pain is frontal or diffuse, radiating to the neck, back, and even the lower extremities. Frequently the patient will volunteer that this is by far the worst headache he has ever had. Within minutes a variable degree of mental confusion may exist. Blood in the subarachnoid space causes a chemical meningitis, and the "meningeal signs" include a stiff neck and Kernig's sign (inability to extend the leg with the thigh flexed). Frequently these patients have a mildly elevated temperature, blood pressure, and pulse. The highly variable clinical signs and symptoms following a subarachnoid hemorrhage are in large part due to vascular spasm resulting in brain ischemia, infarct, and cerebral edema.

The diagnosis of subarachnoid hemorrhage is usually strongly suggested by history and physical examination alone, but a spinal tap usually confirms the diagnosis. After 4 to 12 hr xanthochromia of the cerebrospinal fluid is present, and it disappears from 12 to 40 days after hemorrhage.

The cause of a subarachnoid hemorrhage may be suggested by a history of progressive neurological deficit or seizure disorder or by hearing a cranial bruit with a stethoscope. All of these features would suggest an intracranial vascular malformation. At times, aneurysms may be symptomatic before they hemorrhage and cause varied degrees of headache or extraocular paresis by compression of the third cranial nerve. Blood dyscrasias might be suspected by noting easy bruising or prolonged bleeding from lumbar or venipuncture sites. Frequently, further diagnostic evaluation with arteriography is necessary.

As a general rule, unruptured aneurysm does not require surgical intervention. Diagnostic procedures involving unruptured aneurysms should be limited accordingly. Ruptured aneurysm has a mortality of more than 15% following first rupture and more than 40% mortality following second rupture.

Classic Migraine versus Transient Ischemic Attack

The patient with classic migraine can be distinguished from one suffering transient ischemic attacks (TIAs) by the following:

1. The aura in the classic migraineur lasts several minutes to hours, most often followed by severe headache, usually on the contralateral side.

2. There is weakness or numbness in the arms, often with a spread or march quality, which rarely occurs with TIA.

3.   There is a family history of migraine.

4.   The classic migraineur age group is younger than those with TIA.

5.   Associated symptoms include photophobia and vomiting.

Cerebral Vascular Insufficiency

Basilar artery insufficiency can produce ischemia of the brain stem and pain-sensitive structures below the tentorium as well as occipital areas above the tentorium.   Carotid artery insufficiency can produce ischemia above the tentorium, leading to more anterior appreciation of pain.

Basilar artery insufficiency occurs in middle-aged and older individuals.   Slightly less than half of all patients with vertebrobasilar arterial occlusive disease have headaches either with TIAs or evolution of a stem infarct.

Cerebrovascular Disorder

Pain receptors are within walls of large pain-sensitive arteries; small vessels have few pain receptors and produce no headache or rarely cause headache.   Headache with TIA occur in only 25-40% of patients.   The headache begins at the onset of the neural deficit.

Headaches may occur independent of the above major complications and can simulate migraine.   A prolonged aura persisting after the onset of a headache distinguishes it from migraine. The headache of an arteriovenous malformation is always on the same side as the malformation.   A bruit may be audible over the area of malformation.   Contrary to reports in the literature, in our studies headache occurred in about 15% of angiomas before the development of a seizure disorder or a subarachnoid hemorrhage.

The mechanism of the headache is not certain.   The anomaly may predispose to vascular changes resulting in periodic headaches and, at times, aura.

Aneurysms

Aneurysms with subarachnoid hemorrhage are present predominantly in the fifth to seventh decades.   They are found in approximately 2% of all autopsied cases.

The headache of a ruptured aneurysm is dramatically acute and severe frontal or diffuse, radiating to the neck, back, and even the lower extremities. Depending on the extent and location of bleeding, alterations in the level of consciousness and onset of focal deficits may occur insidiously, rapidly, or intermittently.

However, the headache of an unruptured aneurysm, such as one located at the internal carotid-posterior communicating artery, can cause severe persistent frontal or orbital headache owing to irritation of the dura or can cause extraocular paresis by compression of the third cranial nerve. Regardless of the severity of the associated pain, if the pupil is spared at the onset of an isolated oculomotor palsy, the diagnosis is not aneurysm; the problem is medical, and diabetes is the usual underlying cause. The physician must be alert to the signs of tentorial herniation in which the hemiparesis may be contralateral or ipsilateral, the ipsilateral pupil dilates, and the patient becomes comatose, but often with striking fluctuations of awareness. A CAT scan will visualize the clot, and arteriography shows displacement of cerebral arteries.

Brain Abscess

Signs and symptoms of brain abscess are those of an intracranial expanding lesion. Cerebral edema is prominent in the overall pathophysiology; consequently, headache, nausea, vomiting, and convulsions are early symptoms.

Brain abscesses commonly originate from active or acute bacterial infections involving extracranial sites. A brain abscess may also originate from extracranial fungal and parasitic infections.

Ancillary diagnostic procedures, if positive, can expedite early diagnosis and prompt treatment. These procedures are: a chest x-ray showing a lung abscess, an electroencephalogram showing characteristic focal high-voltage waves, a brain scan demonstrating the presence of one or more foci, or an arteriogram showing an avascular mass.

Arteriovenous Malformations

Arteriovenous malformations are developmental malformations, complex arteriovenous communications varying in size from a mass of tortuous vessels occupying most of one cerebral hemiphere to barely visible blemishes which may involve any part of the brain. Although such malformations may be present at birth, first symptoms may not occur until adolescence or early adult life or may not occur at all. The general symptomatology attains a degree of clinical significance depending on the major neurological complications associated with or caused by the malformation. Three such major complications are subarachnoid hemorrhage, seizure disorder, and progressive neurological deficits.

Diagnosis of an intracranial mass cannot be made on the basis of headache characteristics alone; evaluation of other symptoms and findings found on neurologic examination and the results of ancillary studies are needed for diagnosis.

Pseudotumor Cerebri

Pseudotumor cerebri is a syndrome clinically manifest as headache, papilledema, and diminution of visual acuity. The headache is nonspecific, usually intermittent, and not a constant feature. It is usually present for several weeks to several months before medical attention is sought. Frequently noted as part of the syndrome is the high incidence in young, obese females with menstrual irregularities. However, causes other than ovarian dysfunction are known and include Addison's disease, Cushing's disease, adrenocorticosteroid therapy or withdrawal, hypoparathyroidism, pregnancy, menarche, use of contraceptive drugs, vitamin A abuse, tetracycline use in infants, and intracranial venous sinus thrombosis. The mechanism seems to be that of cerebral swelling causing traction on pain-sensitive structures.

Subdural Hematomas

Subdural hematomas represent the accumulation of blood within the subdural space overlying the cerebral convexities and are closely associated with trauma in the acute and chronic types. There are no characteristic symptoms which will serve to differentiate an acute subdural hematoma from cerebral contusion or laceration. The chronic variety may occur after trivial or closed-head trauma. Headache is a prominent feature of subdural hematoma, although this complaint may be difficult to elicit if the patient is admitted in a confused state. Other symptoms include drowsiness, slowness in thinking, confusion, and occasional agitation, all of which progressively worsen. Focal and lateralizing signs are late and tend to be less prominent than disturbance of consciousness, which may be of a fluctuating nature. In the subacute and chronic types of subdural hematoma, the clinical manifestations are those of a progressive supratentorial mass, which may be characterized by hemiparesis, focal seizures, and choked discs.

Brain Tumors

The headache associated with a lesion in the pituitary fossa is often of a frontal and bitemporal bursting character. The mechanism is of pressure on the diaphragm sella or traction on retro-orbital major basilar vessels. Pain related to a cerebropontine angle lesion is often felt behind the ear.

In tumors occurring in the posterior fossa, headache referred to the occipital and nuchal region is a prominent early sign. These tumors may make their presence known early by obstructing the fourth ventricle. In the presence of increased intracranial pressure, localization of the headache is of little value. Brain stem compression may cause somnolence and vomiting. Even though intracranial pressure may be very high in these patients, they still may not have papilledema, since it can take 24 to 72 hr to reflect the increased pressure at the optic nerve head.

The tumor headache is usually described as paroxysmal, with sudden onset, reaching full intensity in seconds and persisting for minutes or hours, and disappearing abruptly.

Colloid cysts of the third ventricle, tumors of lateral ventricles, and craniopharyngiomas and pinealomas are characterized by bifrontal or generalized pain, usually high intensity and are associated with loss of consciousness and vomiting; transient amaurosis or drop attacks may also be associated.

Glioma and large infiltrating tumors can extend throughout one hemisphere without headache because the position of the large vessels may remain undisturbed.

Meningiomas which compress the brain from the outside are likely to cause seizures, focal symptoms, progressive impairment of intellectual function, and so forth before they produce headache.

Headaches associated with metastatic tumors to the brain can be deceptive. While headache is one of the most common associated manifestations, it is not necessarily constant or severe. Headache is a common early symptom with carcinomatosis of the meninges and may be the presenting symptom for several months before dementia and other symptoms occur.

Chapter 8

Facial Pain

There is not one unifying factor for all types of facial pain. The diagnosis and treatment of facial pain conditions have been an enigma to the practicing physician. Facial pain can occur most often in paroxysmal attacks, and we define these cases as a form of neuralgia. We will also describe the other causes of facial pain.

Trigeminal Neuralgia

Trigeminal neuralgia (tic douloureux) is an episodic, recurrent unilateral pain syndrome which occurs in the elderly. It rarely begins before the age of 50 unless it is symptomatic of under-lying neurological pathology, such as multiple sclerosis. The syndrome shows a preference for women, with the female-to-male ratio being 2:1. The pain is more common on the right side of the face. Bilateral occurrence is uncommon, and there is no familial relationship. The pain is of high intensity and par-ticularly affects trigger zones, which are areas of increased sensitivity on the face and particularly above the naris and mouth, which set off the attacks when they are stimulated, often by tri-vial sensations.

The patient with tic douloureux will avoid washing his face, shav-ing, chewing, or any other maneuver which will stimulate the trigger zones and cause the pain. This avoidance mechanism is a valuable clue in making the diagnosis. Characteristically, a woman will carefully apply her makeup except in the area where the trigger zone exists. Many of these people, because of the trigger zone's location in the oral cavity, will lose a great deal of weight.

Its distribution most often affects the second or third division of the fifth nerve, spreading only late in the disease to the first di-vision. The pain is characteristic of short, sharp, momentary bursts, like electric shocks or a rapid repeating rifle. It is usu-ally excruciating and so severe as to cause the patient to cry out or twitch.   Periods of complete relief are interrupted by attacks caused by exciting the trigger zones.   Since the pain is reflex response to stimulus, it rarely disturbs the sleep of the patient.

A cause has not been proven for trigeminal neuralgia.   Some researchers have blamed a compression of the Gasserian ganglion by the internal carotid artery in the middle cranial fossa.   A degenerative process and a latent virus have also been incriminated.

Anticonvulsants are the drugs of choice in treating trigeminal neuralgia.   They reduce the sensitivity of trigger zones and relieve the pain, often dramatically within hours after beginning therapy.   The drug of choice is phenytoin sodium, up to 400 mg/ day.   Drug blood levels and complete blood counts should be monitored.   If this is not well tolerated, the treatment that should be considered is carbamazepine 200 mg increasing up to 800 to 1200 mg/day.   A combination treatment of phenytoin with carbamazepine may be of some help.   If there is no response, chlorphenesin 400 mg t. i. d. or q. i. d. may be added to the treatment regimen.

Some newer studies have shown that the addition of baclofen to either phenytoin or carbamazepine may be of some help, starting with doses of 10 mg t. i. d. and increasing to a maximum of 80 mg/day.

Surgical intervention becomes essential only if drug treatment fails or when effective dosages cause uncomfortable side effects. Methods of treatment include local alcohol injections, if the pain is confined to a single nerve branch, and thermocoagulation of the nerve fibers of the appropriate division within the Gasserian ganglion through stereotactic control.   This method usually produces excellent results.   The risk of anesthesia of the face or of the cornea is greatly reduced, compared with the injection of the ganglion itself or a division of the sensory tract of the fifth nerve in the midbrain.

The Jannetta procedure has recently been extensively publicized. This comprises an exploration of the posterior fossa and a decompression of the nerve at its point of entry into the pons. This method has been suggested as a form of treatment in intractable cases.   Doctor Jannetta has found that the nerve is compressed by the superior cerebellar artery.[6]   Protection of the nerve with a foam rubber pad from the irritant effect of the redundant arterial loops produces relief from pain in Jannetta's series of cases.

Glossopharyngeal Neuralgia

Rarely, patients will present with a neuralgia affecting the ninth
cranial nerve or the glossopharyngeal nerve. The pain of glossopharyngeal neuralgia is intermittent, severe, and usually described as occurring in the ipsilateral tonsillar fossa, the outer
ear, the back of the tongue, or the angle of the jaw. The patient
indicates that the attacks are induced by coughing, talking,
or swallowing.

The treatment is similar to that of trigeminal neuralgia. There
are some surgical treatments which are rarely needed: (1) avul-
sion of the nerve in the neck, which is simple and frequently
successful; and (2) division of the nerve in the posterior fossa
together with the upper two rootlets of the vagus, as the pain of
the attacks frequently spills over into the vagal sensory distribution due to connecting branches between the two cranial nerves.

Postherpetic Neuralgia

This is a complication of herpes zoster of the face and head. It
occurs most frequently in the elderly.   Close to 20% of the
patients have involvement of the Gasserian ganglion.   The ophthalmic division of the nerve is affected in the remaining cases.
The geniculate ganglion is rarely infected, producing a herp-
etic rash in the external auditory canal with facial palsy (Ramsay-
Hunt syndrome).

The pain of herpes zoster is steady and sustained, and usually
regresses within 2 to 3 weeks.   However, it may persist for
months or years.   The pain is almost always unilateral and has
been described as burning and aching.   The diagnosis presents
little difficulty, as the scars of eruption are too obvious to be
missed.   There are often trophic changes to the skin following
this disorder.   In the majority of cases, the pain tends to disappear within 18 months but can be persistent for the patient's
entire lifetime.

Some physicians initiate treatment with corticosteroids as soon
as the diagnosis is made, and this may be of some help.   The
starting dose is usually prednisone 60 mg daily in divided doses,
gradually decreasing the dose after one week, so that the treatment may be stopped by the end of the third week.   This method
of treatment will reduce the pain of the attack and prevent residual pain.   The use of tricyclic antidepressants is considered
once the diagnosis of postherpetic neuralgia is established. Amitryptiline is the drug of choice, and since these patients are

usually elderly, the dosage should be cautiously increased. The initial dose of 25 mg at night would be gradually increased up to 100 to 150 mg. A phenothiazine, perphenazine, or thioridazine may be considered along with this form of treatment, and the combination may be more successful.

Temporomandibular Joint (TMJ) Dysfunction

This diagnosis is probably one of the most overused terms relating to head pain. The symptoms of TMJ disease consist of localized facial pain, limitation of motion of the jaw, muscle tenderness, and joint crepitus. X-rays of the joint are particularly normal. The pain is situated in front of and behind the ear on the affected side, but may radiate over the cheek and face. There may be a sensation of blockage in the ear. Evidence of hearing loss, damage to the cranial nerves, migraine, cluster headaches, or Meniere's disease have no relationships to temporomandibular joint disease, as is advocated by many dental practitioners.

The treatment of choice is focused on the relief of the muscle spasm, such as simple tranquilizers, muscle relaxants, or biofeedback. Placebo effects are very evident in this condition. Moist heat and massage are also helpful. In some cases, dental splints may be of help. Extensive reconstructions of the mouth are usually not indicated or helpful.

Lower-Half Headache (Facial Migraine)

In this condition, a patient exhibits migrainelike symptoms only affecting the face area below the eye, over the nostril, cheek, and upper jaw. The pain is usually unilateral and of a throbbing nature and has symptoms commonly associated with migraine, such as nausea and vomiting. A family history of migraine usually present. The treatment is similar to that of migraine.

Nasopharyngeal Carcinoma

Those treating facial pain should be aware that these patients should have a thorough workup if they have been unresponsive to treatment by the otolaryngologist. Many cases resembling lower facial migraine or other conditions are actually due to an undiagnosed nasopharyngeal carcinoma.

Atypical Facial Pain

This pain exhibits itself over the second division of the trigeminal nerve, usually lasting hours or days, and is described as constantly present. It may spread across the midline and be bilateral. A typical patient is a woman who is middle-aged, showing signs of anxiety and depression. Atypical facial pain is difficult to diagnose as it lacks definitive criteria, but must be mentioned as a syndrome that has been observed.

There is no consistent treatment for atypical facial pain. However, the drugs of choice are the tricyclic antidepressants. Amitriptyline in particular has helped with an initial dose of 25 mg, increasing the dose gradually because of the age of the patient. Combining it with thioridazine 25 mg t. i. d. may further enhance the action. Psychiatric treatment may be indicated in these cases.

Carotidynia

There are two varieties of carotidynia. The first involves acute onset in young or middle-aged adults in which the pain persists for an average of 11 days and does not usually recur. The pain may radiate to the side of the face in about half of the cases. Tenderness is maximal over the carotid bifurcation, and the patient may have some accompanying nasal blockage and lacrimation. It is probably viral in origin, and the treatment is purely symptomatic.

The second form of carotidynia may occur at any time in life. It is described symptomatically as attacks lasting a few minutes to hours, often with an accompanying throbbing headache. A very prominent symptom common to this disorder is tenderness over the carotid artery. The acute attacks will respond to ergotamine tartrate, and the chronic occurrence of the disease, if prevalent, does respond to treatment with methysergide or propranolol. On physical examination, there may be a tenderness and throbbing and often a dilated carotid artery.

Chapter 9

Headache Due to Eye, Ear, Nose, and Dental Disease

Headaches Due to Eye Disease

Ocular headache localized or involving the eye is common. Photophobia is a frequent occurrence in patients with headache. However, pain and photophobia are rarely caused by disease states of the eye, eye muscles, or optic nerves. Several sections of the eye are pain-sensitive, and the pain sensations are transported by the ophthalmic division of the fifth cranial nerve. Specifically, the conjunctiva and the cornea are clearly pain-sensitive structures. Pain can result from stimulation of the iris and extraocular muscles by traction. Increased intraocular pressure will also precipitate pain.

If pain is triggered by injury or inflammation of the conjunctiva, it is usually of mild to moderate intensity and may be described as burning or aching. The amount of conjunctival injection will facilitate the diagnosis.

Pain due to a corneal abrasion, keratitis, is severe and sustained. It is usually associated with marked photophobia, and a blepharospasm is present. The pain due to increased intraocular pressure is usually localized to the eyeball itself. As the pressure increases, it may involve the entire distribution of the fifth cranial nerve. This pain may be associated with nausea and vomiting. Chronic glaucoma may cause a slight pressure-like sensation, but severe pain is usually caused by acute glaucoma.

Headaches resulting from intraocular inflammatory states, such as uveitis, are commonly associated with normal intraocular pressure and are detected by the presence of inflammatory cells when examined with a slit-lamp microscope. The pain may be severe and throbbing and is localized to the eye and its associated structures. The eye is tender and the pupil may appear small and slightly reactive, secondary to spasm of the iris.

Contrary to common belief, errors in refraction and muscle imbalance are not frequent causes of headache.   When these problems are associated with headache, the visual defect is usually
obvious and the patient will complain of visual difficulties.   If
headaches result from errors in refraction and muscle balance,
the pain will start in and around the eyes and infrequently involves the frontal and occipital areas of the head.   The pain will
be throbbing or nonthrobbing. These headaches will occur following prolonged use of the eyes— in particular, close work and
working in poorly lighted areas.   The pain will usually be relieved by a brief rest period for the eyes.   Hyperopia and astigmatism are refractive errors and can result in an occasional
headache.   Although some of the pain is exhibited by individuals
with refractive errors and extraocular imbalance, much of the
pain may be attributed to sustained contraction of the frontal,
occipital, and neck muscles.   The treatment usually consists
of correction of the errors in refraction and muscle imbalance.

The neuritis which occurs with multiple sclerosis may produce
head pain with an orbital distribution.   It is usually of mild to
moderate intensity, accentuated by head movements.

Headaches Due to Aural Disease

The ear is a common site for referred head pain, although pain
may result from direct involvement of the ear itself.   Pain at
the ear is often referred from remote areas.

Acute otitis externa, acute otitis media, and serous otitis media
may result in ear pain.   Chronic ear infections rarely cause
pain.   If a middle ear infection is present, the rupture of the
tympanic membrane will usually relieve the pain.

Many patients complaining of ear pain will show no evidence of
pathology in the ear canals or the middle ear.   This is usually
due to referred pain because of pathology elsewhere. The auriculo-
temporal branch of the fifth cranial nerve may refer pain to the
ear from the teeth, sinuses, temporomandibular joint, or naso-
pharynx.   Migraine attacks will often manifest as ear pain.

Headaches Due to Nose and Sinus Disease

Diseases of the paranasal sinuses and the nose are frequently
implicated as the cause of headache.   However, they rarely induce recurrent headache problems.   The general population, as
well as physicians, have been brainwashed by mass media ad-
vertising to believe that chronic sinus disease is a cause
of headache. When sinus disease is the provocative factor, the diagnosis is easily formulated.

Acute sinus disease causes pain radiating over the frontal regions while maxillary sinusitis usually produces pain over the maxillary region. Diseases of the ethmoid and sphenoid sinuses usually produce pain behind the eyes and over the vertex.

The pain of diseases affecting the paranasal sinuses is dull, aching, and nonpulsating. It may be aggravated by jarring. In order for sinus disease to cause a headache, there must be an obstruction of the sinus with a pus-producing inflammation. The mucosa covering the approach to the paranasal sinuses has been observed to be the most pain-sensitive of the nasal and sinus structures. However, the mucosa lining the sinuses themselves are relatively insensitive to pain. Inflammation and enlargement of the turbinates and superior nasal surfaces are the cause of most of the pain emanating from the nasal and paranasal sinuses. It should be reiterated that there must be an elevated temperature and an obstruction to cause sinus or paranasal disease. The treatment consists of decongestants, both oral and nasal, and antibiotics.

Headaches Due to Dental Disease

Dental disease is a rare cause of headache. The painful sensation of dental disease is usually transmitted by the second and third divisions of the fifth cranial nerve. These divisions enter the pulp and the apex of the tooth. The pain experienced by individuals with dental disease is described as burning and aching in quality. Usually, the pain is first localized to a tooth. It may radiate chronically to other structures innervated by the same divisions of the fifth cranial nerve. Secondary pain in the head and neck may result from sustained muscle contraction in the region of the dental pain. The goal of treatment is focused on correcting the primary dental problem. (Temporomandibular joint disease has been discussed in Chapter 8 on facial pain.)

Chapter 10

Temporal Arteritis

Temporal arteritis is an inflammatory condition of undetermined cause. It usually affects branches of the carotid artery and rarely if ever occurs in patients before the age of 55. It is more prevalent in women. If the condition is diagnosed and treated before it has progressed, serious complications such as blindness can be avoided. The important clue in diagnosing the case is headache of recent onset in a patient over the age of 55. There will not be a chronic history of headache.

Temporal arteritis often exhibits symptoms of systemic disturbance such as weight loss, night sweating, aching of the joints, and fever. It is often part of a syndrome known as "polymyalgia rheumatica. " Many of the patients will have a history suggestive of rheumatoid arthritis or frequent complaints of muscle pains.

Patients rarely seek medical care before the onset of their headache symptoms. Headache is probably the major and most prominent symptom and may be quite severe. The pain is often unilateral but can be bilateral, and is easily differentiated from the simple tension or muscle contraction headache the patient may have suffered previously. The pain will be localized over one temple and will be described as intense, boring, and occasionally stabbing along the course of the temporal vessel. The patient may have difficulty sleeping and may sit up in bed for an entire night because the pain is so intense.

Because of anatomical considerations of the temporal artery, the patient will exhibit discomfort on opening the mouth and pain and stiffness in the region of the temporomandibular joint. Excessive chewing may cause an intermittent claudication of the jaw. Many patients develop wasting and weight loss due to difficulty in chewing. In several cases, patients have been prescribed bite plates and have had excessive mouth reconstruction because of the failure of the physician or dentist to recognize this condition. If the vessels supplying the central nervous system are involved, there may be other symptoms such as delirium, confusion, and eighth nerve involvement. Red nodules over the temporal region are sometimes noted, and the patient may refer to them as varicose veins. There may be tenderness over the temporal artery on examination and the pulsations may be diminished or absent. When rolled beneath the temporal fossa, there may be a feeling of a stringlike hardness to the temporal artery in extremely thin patients. This is not a normal or frequent finding.

An early diagnosis is important in temporal arteritis to prevent patients from developing visual symptoms. This can occur from several weeks to 5 or more months after symptoms of the disease are paramount. The visual symptoms are caused by a decrease in the blood supply to the optic nerve. The patients may also feel symptoms of ophthalmoplegia, diplopia, ptosis, and other evidence of ocular motor paralysis. The visual disturbances due to arteritis of the posterior ciliary arteries and other branches of the ophthalmic artery with the resultant ischemia of the optic nerve develops in about 50% of the untreated patients with the disease. In many of these patients, transient visual blurring may precede their blindness.

The one specific diagnostic test is a sedimentation rate by Westergen method. In any patient over the age of 55 who develops headache for the first time, this is a mandatory procedure. Almost invariably the sedimentation rate is above normal, although on occasion it can be within normal limits. Most often, it is above 60 mm/hr. In a patient with a markedly increased sedimentation rate and where there is a suspicion of temporal arteritis, a biopsy is essential. In blood tests, these patients also exhibit a hypochromic anemia. Biopsy of the superficial temporal artery shows almost complete obliteration of the lumen with some recanalization. High-powered microscopy reveals infiltration with lymphocytes, plasma cells, and giant cells and fragmentation of the elastica.

The clinical picture of temporal arteritis may be so bizarre that continuous clinical vigilance is necessary to assure early diagnosis and treatment and thus prevention of serious complications. The disease may be suspected even though biopsy is normal. Treatment should be implemented because the complications of the disease can be so catastrophic.

Treatment of Arteritis

The treatment of choice is the corticosteroids, giving from 60 to 80 mg of prednisone immediately upon diagnosis. Treatment should be continued while gradually reducing the levels of prednisone for 6 to 8 months, since this length of time has been known to elapse between the onset of headache and the visual impairment. Once the visual impairment has occurred, steroid therapy is of little value. The dose of prednisone should be monitored by the sedimentation rate and the symptoms. Patients should be seen quite often. If they have a return of the headache or constitutional symptoms, the amount of steroids should be increased.

Some patients have been known to improve without therapy after biopsy, but this is a rare occurrence and should not be the method of choice. In most cases, the disease resolves 6 to 8 months after therapy, and the patients will have no further recurrence.

Chapter 11

Management of Post-traumatic Headache

The post-traumatic headache is a prominent part of a syndrome
previously described as the postconcussion syndrome. This
syndrome includes headache, vertigo, memory loss, emotional
lability, and poor powers of concentration following an open or
closed head injury. Children may manifest marked personality
changes such as aggressiveness, hyperkinesis, learning disability, and enuresis in addition to the symptoms listed above.
Several studies set the incidence of one or more of these symptoms at 30-80%.

It is common for the head-injured patient to complain, spontaneously or when questioned, of pain which lasts hours or days,
and then resolves. Brenner and Friedman in 1944, [7, 9] and
Jacobsen in 1969[8], studied a group of patients with minor closed
head injuries and found that approximately 94% experienced pain
within 24 hr, while only 6% noted the onset of headache for several days or weeks past the initial event.

Chronic post-traumatic headache is distinguished by a duration of
2 months or longer. The incidence of development of chronic
post-traumatic headache is 30-50% in several series. In attempts
to define which factors predict the occurence of chronic headache, Brenner in 1944 and Kay in 1971[10] found no correlation
with the presence of the following factors: loss of consciousness
of variable duration; posttraumatic amnesia; EEG abnormalities
(up to 7 days past event); skull fracture; and blood in cerebrospinal fluid. Thus, more severe head injuries would not
cause chronic headache. Chronic discomfort following neuro-
surgical procedures, such as craniotomy, is rare. Some authors'
observations, however, indicate that the development of chronic
headache occurs rarely without provocation by trauma, associated disorientation, or amnesia. The physician should be
aware that even minor head trauma can be associated with sub-
sequent intractable pain.

In understanding which injuries are more likely to result in chronic post-traumatic headache, one must consider the background of the patient and the circumstances of injury.   Sheeley in 1980[11] noted that psychiatric surveys of general populations routinely reveal undiagnosed and unrecognized psychiatric disorders. Although some patients with preexisting psychiatric disturbances are prone to the development of symptoms following head injury, this is not a general rule.   The anxious, nervous, or depressed patient presents more complaints over a longer period of time. Hysterical patients may exaggerate symptoms.   Response to therapy for the headache is suboptimal; recovery may be abnormally prolonged until the underlying emotional disorder is recognized and treated.

Pending litigation has also been shown to influence a patient's response to head injury.   Taylor in 1967[12] demonstrated a positive correlation between the number of symptoms and pending litigation in a group of patients with similar injuries. Authors such as Miller in 1961[13] have shown that earlier resolution of legal and financial problems leads to faster recovery.   However, many authors (Critchley et al.[14]) feel that the severity, frequency, or residual nature of head pain is not dependent on compensation. This is also the belief of the authors.

It is apparent that no simple approach to the patient with chronic post-traumatic headache is available. One must understand the nature of the injury and the resulting headache, as well as the complexity of the patient's response to his injury. The physician must be cognizant of both organic and psychological factors.

It is generally accepted that there are at least four different kinds of chronic post-traumatic headache. Each has a proposed mechanism and characteristic manifestation.   Keep in mind that coexistence of these headache types is common.

Type I

The most frequently observed post-traumatic headache is essentially indistinguishable from the muscle contraction or tension headache.   In one series by Simon and Wolf.[15] it accounted for 70% of the post-traumatic headache studied.   This headache is a constant, dull, nonthrobbing pressure sensation which may be focal or diffuse.   The patient may delineate a band, tightened about one area of the head.   EMG studies of the focal muscles have demonstrated increased activity with head pain.   With this discomfort, vertigo, lightheadedness, and giddiness may be experienced.   Anxiety, malaise, and fatigue may also be prominent features. Pain generation may be secondary to sustained muscular contraction plus buildup of metabolites. Some authors postulate that a central defect in muscle tone regulation, involving the gamma afferent system, occurs with head injury.

The antidepressant amitriptyline is a successful therapeutic modality for the post-traumatic headache. Initial doses of 25-75 mg before bedtime are recommended. Response may be titrated to anticholinergic side effects. With disappearance of the dry mouth (commonly at 4-6 weeks) and headache recurrence, the dosage may be incrementally increased up to 250 mg. If side effects are intolerable or treatment failure occurs, desipramine may work well. After several months of response (absence or infrequent headaches), the medication may be tapered slowly. Without recurrence or exacerbation, it can sometimes be completely withdrawn.

Type II

In the series described earlier, 14% of chronic post-traumatic headaches are described as a local area of tenderness and pain. A palpable and tender scar may be present. The type II headache occurs one to three times per week and may last for hours. It is usually a focal, mild to moderate throbbing pain which may be accompanied by nausea and photophobia. Local sensory nerve entrapment or incomplete nerve disruption may produce the pain. There may be a focal myositis, fibrositis, or periostitis.

Treatment with local injections of up to 7-8 cc of 1% xylocaine may produce immediate relief. If repeated injections are necessary, a prolonged response may result from the addition of 1.5 cc of dexamethasone to the xylocaine.

This headache may coexist with the type I headache described. Successful treatment could depend upon resolution of the sustained muscular contraction. Surgical nerve or ligament release may be required in some cases, such as occipital nerve decompression for refractory occipital neuralgia.

Type III

Post-traumatic migraine was observed in 6% of a group studied by Simon and Wolf. [15] Patients complained of severe, unilateral throbbing pain. Scotomata may precede these attacks, which occur weekly, and can last from minutes to days. Associated photophobia, nausea, and occasional emesis are also observed. Malaise and fatigue may be prominent factors. Dilated, palpable

extracranial vessels are described. Patients may find relief
from focal pressure or application of ice. Without relief, these
headaches can be incapacitating.

Migraines may be present in family members. A study of Haas,
et al.[16] of 25 children with juvenile head trauma syndrome
demonstrated that attacks of cortical blindness, hemiparesis,
somnolence, and brain stem dysfunction following minor head
trauma were identical to juvenile classical migraine. Recur-
rences with or without repeated head injury were seen. Of note,
15 of these 25 children ($\leqslant$ 14 years) had positive family histories
for migraine. There was also a 12% incidence of transient focal
neurologic abnormalities with migraine in family members.

Autonomic dysfunction with vasomotor instability is believed to
cause post-traumatic migraine. Oldendorf and Kitano in 1967[17]
demonstrated increased cerebral circulation time with post-
traumatic symptoms. The flow was normal without the presence of a headache. Regulation of precapillary arterioles may
be abnormal. Some authors have proposed that sustained muscular contraction may directly affect extracerebral vasculature.
Studies with intravenous histamine, shown to dilate intracerebral vessels, have demonstrated reproduction of typical symptoms in patients with chronic post-traumatic headache.

Propranolol, 20-80 mg, has been used successfully in the prophylaxis of some post-traumatic headaches. Treatment with 25-
50 mg of amitriptyline at bedtime may also decrease recurrence of headache. In children, Periactin (cyproheptadine) used
before bedtime has been extremely useful in prevention. These
posttraumatic migraines may also respond to ergots. Changes
in diet or sleep pattern, biofeedback, and other modalities
frequently used in migraine treatment may be indicated in
these situations.

Type IV

In 1975, Vijayan and Dreyfus[18] described traumatic dysautonomic cephalalgia in five patients with injury to the anterior tri-
angle of the neck. Blunt, nonlacerating, or stretch injuries were
incurred. These patients had unilateral (ipsilateral to injury)
throbbing head pain with excessive sweating and pupillary dilation. Photophobia, visual blurring, and nausea accompanied
the headache. Between attacks, unilateral miosis and ptosis
occurred in four of five patients. Pharmacologic studies suggested partial sympathectomy. There was no response to ergots.
Beta-sympathetic overactivity is suggested as the cause of this
syndrome. These patients responded well to propranolol, 80 mg
daily.

Some post-traumatic headaches can be caused by blood in the extradural, subdural, or subarachnoid space. Fibrous adhesions in pain-sensitive areas may be involved. Exacerbation with movement, coughing, or sneezing is frequent, but is not included in diagnostic criteria for this problem. Patients with types I, II, or III chronic posttraumatic headache may have similar components. These headaches commonly disappear after a few days or weeks.

Pain referred to the head from cervical pathology may be observed similarly to whiplash injuries. Damaged muscle, ligaments, discs, bones, or nerve roots may be the origin of pain. The pain may be focal or suboccipital-occipital or may spread to involve all areas. Associated neck and scalp muscular contraction could induce pain or exacerbate preexisting pain. Treatment with a neck brace, physical therapy, and/or local steroid injections for nerve root problems may be considered. If nerve entrapment is evident, surgical release may be necessary.

It must be stressed that these four types of headache frequently coexist. This may indicate similar pathogenesis, or one type of headache may induce or exacerbate another type. Elimination of one type may facilitate control of another.

The effect of psychological factors on the development of post-traumatic syndrome and headache must be emphasized. The physician should attempt to discern as much as possible about the patient's constitution and personality. He should determine the circumstances of the injury and the possibility of pending litigation. This information will aid in differentiating the psychological from the organic nature of the problem.

It has been demonstrated that the organic factors involved are supported by the changes in total or regional blood flow. Cortical dysfunction manifested by slower visual evoked response times and decreased informational processing has been documented in previous patients with head injury. Abnormalities of norepinephrine/serotonin limbic and frontotemporal pathways have been noted. Vasomotor instability secondary to autonomic dysfunction may be an important provocative factor in vascular headaches.

Prognosis to therapy is dependent on a number of poorly defined factors. Jacobson,[8] in a study of 46 patients with minor head injury, found that the majority of patients eventually lost their headaches within 2 months. These headaches did not fit the definition of chronicity. He stated that patients with headaches over a 4-year period were unlikely to respond to therapy. Studies such as Kelley's in 1975[19] show a statistically significant decrease in the duration of disability from post-traumatic headache with a particularly positive physician-patient interaction. This involved daily visits, full explanation of the injury and the headache, encouragement for early ambulation, and early physical therapy.

Recently, one of the authors has observed that the use of the antiinflammatory drugs— in particular, indomethacin— has been effective in some post-traumatic headache patients. Successful management of the chronic post-traumatic headache depends upon the physician's awareness of headache patterns and his sensitivity to the intricacies of human nature.

The pediatrician and the family practicioner will see many children presenting the complaint of headache. It is difficult for the
physician to determine if the cause of the headache is organic
or "psychogenic. " A careful history is the key to the diagnosis.
This should be completed with a thorough physical and neurological examination. Appropriate testing should be considered in
order to rule out an organic illness. Less than 8% of all children with headache problems will have an organic cause to
their headaches.

In children, the incidence of headache has been estimated between 2. 5% and 35%. As the child ages, especially the female
patient at menarche, the headaches become more frequent.

As stated previously, the headache history is the most important
key to the diagnosis. The child should be carefully questioned
and possibly the parents should be interviewed. Usually the
child alone can provide sufficient information the the examin-
ing physician.

During the physical examination, vital signs may give a clue to
the underlying cause of the headache problem. Fever, for example, is a definitive symptom of an infectious process. If the
blood pressure is elevated in the upper extremities, it should
also be checked in the lower extremities to rule out coarctation
of the aorta. All organs should be checked due to their possible
relationship to the child's headaches. (Please review Chapter 3.)

When considering diagnostic testing, it should be noted that the
EEG is of limited value in the assessment of children with headaches, except in those patients with a coexisting epilepsy or an
epileptic equivalent. Computerized axial tomography (CAT scan)
is probably the most definitive diagnostic tool in providing information on a wide variety of disorders, including brain tumors,
congenital arteriovenous malformations, intracranial infections,

trauma, and degenerative vascular disease. More sophisticated tests such as arteriography or pneumoencephalography are usually not indicated. (See Chapter 3.)

Acute Organic Headache Syndromes

Astigmatism, refractive errors, and squint are frequently suspected to be causes of headaches in children, but this occurs rather infrequently. When eyesight is associated with the headaches, it is usually related to reading, watching television, and schoolwork. Headaches due to eyesight difficulties usually occur in the late afternoon or evening. These headaches can often be relieved by corrective reading glasses. Glaucoma is very rare in children.

Headache may be a nonspecific symptom of any type of fever or infection. Increased temperature causes a vasodilation with resulting headache. Sinusitis, although it was once considered by most physicians and patients to be a frequent cause of head pain, is a rare cause of headache. If acute sinusitis is present, it is accompanied by fever, persistent rhinorrhea, cough, evidence of ear infection, and allergy. Physical examination reveals a suppurative discharge from the nose or evidence of nasal blockage. X-ray examination will also note evidence of an infection.

Trauma can be a frequent cause of headache in children and may occur in two forms. The pain may localize at the area of trauma and be related to nerve and tissue injury at the site. The pain may be persistent for a few days, weeks, or months. Skull fractures or brain injuries should be ruled out. Usually reassuring the patient as well as giving analgesics and the passage of time will promote improvement. The second form of trauma-related headache is the development of a postconcussion syndrome. In this disorder, the headache may be associated with a sleep disturbance, restlessness, personality change, memory difficulties, dizziness, and school problems. The prognosis in these cases is not encouraging, but the use of antidepressants, such as protryptiline (Vivactil), has been found helpful in some of these patients.

Chronic or Progressive Organic Headache Syndromes

Chronic, progressive headaches due to organic causes are primarily due to increased intracranial pressure. Traction on the large arteries and veins induces pain. Increased intracranial pressure causes headaches, nausea, vomiting, ataxia, loss of strength, seizures, extreme lethargy, or personality and handwriting changes.

The headache due to a brain tumor usually increases in intensity and never regresses.   The site of the pain is not of localizing value, but exertion such as coughing, straining for a bowel movement, running, or any other activity which increases the intracranial pressure will intensify the pain.   In a young child, restlessness and irritability may be the only signs of head pain.

Pseudotumor cerebri is increased intracranial pressure without any evidence of obstruction to the cerebral spinal fluid. The most common signs are a choked disc or papilledema and a sixth nerve paralysis.   A CAT scan will not demonstrate a tumor, and the ventricles are normal size.   However, in these cases a lumbar puncture is essential and will reveal increased pressure.   The physician should be suspicious in those patients taking tetracycline, excessive amounts of vitamin A, or oral contraceptives or in those patients who are obese or have a hormone or menstrual irregularity.

Hydrocephalus is due to blockage of the spinal fluid circulation or a failure of the fluid to be absorbed properly. The symptoms are of increased intracranial pressure, and the CAT scan demonstrates dilated ventricles.

Since subdural hematomas result from trauma, they are often seen in the battered child syndrome.   The headache resulting from subdural hematomas is often accompanied by seizures and other focal neurological deficits.   Brain abscesses, which were once frequent occurrences, have been almost obliterated by antibiotics used in chronic ear infections.

Vascular Headaches

Cluster headaches occur very rarely in children. It can occur in children as young as eight years old.   The onset of migraine often presents in childhood.   A disturbance in consciousness, accompanied by agitation, may be the significant symptom of migraine in children. It is important for the physician to differentiate these symptoms from an acute mental disturbance, such as encephalopathy or toxic metabolic disorders.

Basilar artery migraine is defined as recurrent attacks of neurological dysfunction affecting the posterior circulation. These episodes occur suddenly and usually disappear completely. The symptoms include confusion, hemiparesis, vertigo, and ataxia. This type of migraine occurs more frequently in females. Its neurological manifestations may be the only indication of the presence of migraine.

Unexplained episodes of motion sickness and cyclic vomiting have been reported in children and may result in dehydration. Many of these cases may be forerunners of migraine symptoms.

In many children, episodes of headache, nausea, and vomiting are considered seizure equivalents. This diagnosis should be reserved for episodes of headache accompanied by states of altered consciousness. To confirm this diagnosis, a history of seizures should be elicited as well as an EEG pattern revealing spike activity. A positive family history of seizures as well as a good response to anticonvulsants will also substantiate this diagnosis. In general, anticonvulsants are of little value in the treatment of migraine in children.

Up to the time of puberty, migraine occurs more frequently in males. At menarche, the ratio changes so that migraine is seen more often in the female. Migraine may be precipitated by many factors, such as: stress, fatigue, trauma, exercise, illness, allergies, diet, oral contraceptives, and menses. The headache is usually unilateral and is throbbing in nature. It is often associated with nausea and vomiting. The frequency will vary, from three per week to one per year, and the duration will range from 30 min to 2 days.

The treatment of migraine in children must be individualized. It will be determined by the frequency of the acute attacks, the presence or absence of an aura, and the age and reliability of the patient. If the attacks are infrequent, the patient should receive sedatives, antiemetics, and analgesics at the time of the severe headache. In the adolescent patient, frequent and infrequent attacks can be treated with ergot compounds, such as Cafergot, if taken at the first sign of the aura or headache, and repeated in 1 half-hour. No more than three doses should be taken in a single day, and the drug should not be repeated in less than 4 days.

In the prophylaxis of migraine in children and adolescents, the drug of choice is cyproheptadine (Periactin). In younger children the dose should be started at 4 mg/day, and with older children up to 12 mg/day. Children unresponsive to this therapy may be treated with propranolol, using 60 to 100 mg daily in divided doses. The contraindications to treatment with propranolol are asthma, insulin-dependent diabetes, cardiac failure, and peripheral vascular disease.

Muscle Contraction Headaches

In children, muscle contraction headaches occur frequently. The patient will describe the pain as diffuse and sometimes bandlike. The headache is not usually associated with nausea and vomiting, but may be accompanied by muscle spasm and tenderness at the neck.

Muscle contraction headache is almost always related to stress situations.   Therefore, a careful inventory of the patient's family and school relationships is indicated.   The parents and the patient should be interviewed together and separately.   Counseling may be indicated, and if the problem is not resolved, the physician should consider a psychiatric consultation. In children, depression can occur, and treatment with an antidepressant such as amitryptiline (Elavil) may be helpful.   The acute pain may be relieved by simple analgesics.

It has been reported that children will respond very well to biofeedback training.   This may be due to the fact that children have not yet learned a pain pattern and can readily utilize biofeedback techniques in relieving the headaches. It should also be noted that children find the techniques easier to learn that adult patients and enjoy using the instrumentation.   Biofeedback is an excellent treatment modality for children in order that they not become dependent on medications.

Chapter 13

Iatrogenic Headache

Confirming a drug as a cause of headache is quite difficult because of the fact that headaches do come from various sources,
including the underlying illness being treated. Fever does produce vasodilation and can cause, as one of its primary symptoms, headache. Thus, it would be improper to incriminate an
antibiotic for a headache which is induced by an infectious or
bacterial disease.

Also, it is difficult to measure the symptoms of headache in people taking drugs. Including patients taking placebos, as many
as 25% of these subjects will report headache as a side effect.
The controlled groups in these studies cause difficulty in assess-
ing headache as a complication of drug therapy. The use of multiple medications will further complicate the study of the possible
adverse effects of a drug. However, the mechanisms by which
drugs can cause headaches include (1) hypertension—through
vasodilation in the head area or through hypertensive encephalopathy; (2) extracranial and intracranial vasodilation—by
the nitrites and nitrates, and occurring without hypertension;
(3) intracranial hypertension—increased intracranial pressure
can cause papilledema, vomiting, and may be induced by certain
antibiotics and anesthetics, and will usually disappear with the
discontinuance of these drugs; and (4) alteration of the biochemical status of the brain, such as the effect of various drugs on
serotonin. Headache can result from variations of the pO_2 and
pCO_2 in the brain area. Low partial pressure of oxygen in the
cerebral tissue can induce severe headache. Increased partial
pressure of carbon dioxide frequently worsens headaches—for
example, the headache which occurs when traveling to a higher
altitude. Biochemical changes which raise the intracranial pressure or cause vasodilation may be potential mechanisms for
headache induction. Peripheral neuropathies caused by drugs
such as digitoxin or hydroxystilbamidine are very difficult
to diagnose.

76

Hypertension

Drugs that suddenly increase blood pressure can induce headache. When the catecholamines (epinephrine, phenylephrine) or similar drugs are given either intravenously or intramuscularly, there may be a sudden increase in blood pressure. The amphetamine-like drugs which replace norepinephrine at the nerve endings can cause similar effects. The hypertensive drugs, through induction of hypersensitivity of peripheral adrenergic receptors, may also cause headaches. The primary ones are guanethidine, bretylium, bethanidine, and debrisoquine. Apresoline and praxosin hydrochloride (Minipress) cause vasodilation and can have headache symptoms as a side effect. Monoamine oxidase inhibitors, when used to treat depression or persistent headache, can interreact with sympathomimetic drugs, foods containing tyramine, or alcoholic beverages and induce a very severe hypertensive crisis, headache, or even stroke in less fortunate individuals. Acute reserpine administration has been reported to precipitate migrainelike headache in susceptible individuals. Some patients will suffer a severe headache when hypertensive drugs are withdrawn abruptly. Patients can experience headache due to rapid withdrawal of clonidine or the beta blockers, and rapid rebound hypertension is the cause of the headache.

Adrenocortical dysfunction is observed in treatment with steroids and sometimes induces headaches. However, the headache that occurs during the withdrawal of these drugs may be due to an adrenal insufficiency.

Ergotamine

The abuse of ergotamine tartrate by patients with migraine does occur. However, ergotism in such patients is uncommon. The clinical picture of ergotism is quite explicit. Initially, copious vomiting occurs. The extremities, commonly the lower extremities, may become pulseless and congested and will change in color. Finally, gangrene may develop and can be accompanied by jaundice and convulsions. The physician must be aware that a patient who has a fever, infection, or liver disease is more prone to ergot reactions.

A common occurrence with the abuse of ergots is what we call a rebound phenomenon. Patients who take ergots on a daily basis will develop a rebound headache on the day they stop the ergots or the following day. This occurrence tends to intensify the use of the drug on a daily basis. The instructions to the patient must be explicit in that the drug should not be repeated in less than 3 to 4 days.

Caffeine

The excessive consumption of coffee, tea, or cola or the excessive intake of caffeine-containing drugs such as Excedrin or
Anacin may result in a throbbing headache caused by vasodilation. Patients taking an excessive amount of caffeine will need
to be slowly tapered off these drugs.

Hangover (Alcohol) Headache

Hangover headache has been attributed to vasodilation. The pain
has been relieved by caffeine and ergotamine preparations. A-
nother type of therapy has been suggested to reduce the frequency and severity of the hangover headache. Using fructose,
30 g, in the form of honey, can increase the rate of alcohol metabolism. Headache due to hangover is a self-limited condition.

Nitrites and Nitrates

Some drugs act directly on the vascular musculature in the head
and induce a vasodilation that leads to headaches. The most
prominent of these drugs are the nitrites and nitrates, such as
drugs used for cardiac purposes—that is, nitroglycerin, amyl
nitrate, and other nitrates. Headaches occuring after the ingestion of hotdogs and cured meats are due to the addition of
nitrites to the foods as a preservative. These compounds are
thought to cause headache by displacing the central amines such
as serotonin from the synoptic nerve endings. Fenfluramine,
parachlorophenylalanine, indomethacin, ibuprofen, ketoprofen,
and alclofenac acid have been implicated. Also, certain drugs
such as the nitrates, the sulfonamides, and aniline compounds
can be hypoxic and cause a headache and also can cause biochemical actions.

There is a marked number of drugs that can increase intracranial pressure. This occurs most often in children. Increased
intracranial pressure usually appears after the prolonged use
of the drugs, which are usually at therapeutic levels. The patients exhibit papilledema, nausea, vomiting, and sometimes a
sixth cranial nerve palsy. Most of these manifestations will
disappear when the drug is withdrawn.

Antibiotics

Antibiotics, primarily nalidixic acid, tetracycline, and ampicil-
lin, have been implicated. Griseofulvin, an antifungal agent, is
another of the causative agents. The use of halothane, ketamine,

and enflurane have also been implicated in this type of disorder. Also, excessive amounts of vitamin A may be a provocative factor.

Birth Control Pills, Estrogens, and Postmenopausal Hormones

It is felt that migraine is a vasomotor disorder, and since estrogens alter vasomotor stability, the use of estrogens may increase the frequency, severity, duration, and complications of migraine. There is an increased incidence of vascular headache in young women using the oral contraceptive pill, as well as an increased incidence of stroke. This incidence is also seen in women taking postmenopausal estrogens. Rarely, the use of estrogens in postmenopausal patients will improve the headaches. However, it is generally best to avoid altering the normal menstrual cycle of women who have migraine or women in the menopausal stages.

Chapter 14

Biofeedback and Its Application to Headache

In the past, the scientific study of behavior has generally been
concerned with the physical aspects of biological organisms.
Human beings have been the primary subject of this research,
and their behavior is the most complex, least understood , and
most interesting. In order to comprehend this complicated being
the objective world of observable phenomena has been used as
the guideline. Study has been limited to external and internal
events which are measurable. Most scientific data regarding
behavior have resulted from observations of individuals reacting
with the external environment.

In our efforts to understand these interactions with the external
environment, the concept of "self" has been ignored. Efforts
at attaining self-awareness have been an important element in
many Eastern cultures for several centuries. These efforts
have been related to a physiological discipline. This has been
illustrated in the philosophies of the yogis, Zen masters, and
other disciples of self-awareness. Many of these disciples will
spend entire lifetimes in order to achieve this total self-awareness.
and physical self-control and search for total harmony with the
external environment.

Origin of Biofeedback Techniques

The discipline of self-awareness has been considered irrelevant
and too exotic for Western culture. Control over autonomic
functions has been considered doubtful, especially by members
of the scientific community. However, recent research has
revealed the definite presence of a biological basis for these
practices. Through this research, the technique of biofeedback
has been developed. Biofeedback allows the subject to gain self-
control by using a mechanical device and therefore complies
with the standards of Western culture. This therapy combines
modern electric technology with ancient Eastern practices and
modern psychology. Various bodily functions, such as heart

rate, blood pressure, temperature, muscle tension, and brain-wave activity, are monitored on complex electric devices. The term "feedback" was coined by the mathematician Norbert Weiner, who defined it as a method of controlling the system by reinserting into it the results of its past performances. In biofeedback, the results are artificially mediated by mechanical detection amplification and display instrumentation rather than being present as an inborn feedback loop in the biological system. It is, simply, a method of teaching a person to control a previously unused or involuntarily controlled function of the body through the use of instrumentation. Biofeedback is usually used to control the autonomic nervous system and thus controls functions such as blood flow, blood pressure, and heartbeat. It also is used to teach a person to control previously unused portions of the motor nervous system. These techniques are based on Pavlovian or classical conditioning. This research led to the development of the theory of operant conditioning which is the basis for instrumental learning or biofeedback techniques. In this technique, a conditioned stimulus is provided along with an opportunity to respond in various ways. The correct response is reinforced or rewarded. After several reinforcements, the conditioned stimulus becomes a signal to the subject to perform the learned response. For humans, the knowledge of their accomplishments is sometimes the only reinforcement needed.

About the time Pavlov was developing his theory of conditioning, Johannes Schultz was devising a mind-body training system termed autogenic training. This was accomplished with the subject directing himself by speaking aloud a series of phrases to help him relax. The physician serves merely as a teacher so that this system would be considered self-regulation. Edmond Jacobson had also developed a method of teaching mind-body control. His system was termed progressive relaxation training and was similar to that of Schultz. Neither of these training systems is popular as a great deal of training is required to obtain any noticeable results.

Biofeedback training relies on these techniques of self-regulation but employs instrumentation to speed-up the process. The most successful application of biofeedback, clinically, has been with the treatment of headache. The concept of using biofeedback and autogenic training in the treatment of migraine was initiated at the Menninger Foundation under Doctor Elmer Green. A volunteer in the biofeedback research program noted she was able to abort a headache at the time she was attempting to increase blood flow in the hand and thus raise her hand temperature.

This incident led to the "hot-hand" theory of migraine therapy developed by Sargent, Green, and Walters. [20] Their staff had observed that local peripheral temperature was directly related to the blood flow in the area.   Using the autogenic phrases of Schultz and a device to monitor the temperature of the hand, the subjects at Menninger were able to elevate the hand temperature and in some cases abort or alleviate a migraine.

While research was being completed at the Menninger Foundation on temperature biofeedback training for migraine therapy, Budzynski, Stoyva, and Adler[21] were developing a technique for deep muscle relaxation through the use of an electromyographic (EMG) monitor.   The subject would hear a tone with a frequency proportional to the EMG level of the muscle.   As the muscle was relaxed the tone would decrease; and conversely, muscle tension would bring about a louder tone.   This technique was used with volunteers with tension headaches.   The subjects were taught to relax the frontalis muscle, and this resulted in a decrease in the frequency and severity of the headaches.

In this combination of autogenic and biofeedback training, the patient becomes involved in the treatment.   This concept is definitely a break with the traditional physician-patient relationship.   Through this training, the patient becomes aware of his internal environment and enables the patient to judge his responses to that environment.   It is the goal of biofeedback training to provide the patient with some degree of voluntary control over physiological functions.

For the physician, choosing the correct modality of biofeedback for the individual patient is essential.   Two methods of biofeedback training are applicable for the patient with vascular headaches.   The patient with classic migraine has a warning preheadache and will be able to utilize temperature training at the first sign of headache.   EMG feedback can provide the patient with vascular headache an ability to relax despite the headache and may decrease the severity and duration of the headache.   Patients with a mixed diagnosis—that is, vascular headaches and muscle contraction headaches—are most successful with a combination of temperature and EMG training.   Those patients with muscle contraction headaches exclusively may be successful with EMG training only.

Biofeedback Procedures

The process of biofeedback training will be detailed according
to procedures employed by Dr. Diamond.   Initial training usually consists of an intensive 4- to 5-week period with follow-up
training dependent on the patient's response to biofeedback.   Local patients are seen twice weekly for 4 weeks while patients
from out of town will initiate biofeedback training with an intensive 2-week period of twice-daily sessions at the clinic facility.
At the end of 4 weeks, each patient is evaluated and is encouraged
to continue twice-daily practice sessions at home.

During the clinic visits, the patient is seated in a dimly lit, quiet
room in a recliner chair.   Patient rooms in the biofeedback facility are not furnished in typical clinical decor.   The focus is
on relaxation and warmth.   The patient is advised to practice
at home in a similar environment.   However, the patient should
be advised that the environment is not essential to success in
utilizing the biofeedback to abort the headache.

A temperature biofeedback trainer machine is leased to each
patient for a period of 4 weeks.   The patient is advised to keep
accurate records of each home practice session, recording his
initial and final temperature readings at each session. Each session consists of 10 min on the monitor with the patient utilizing
the autogenic phrases of Schultz.   These phrases focus on warmth
and relaxation, and the patient is also encouraged to focus on a
warm image — for example, a hot bath, sitting by a fire.   The
following are the autogenic phrases of Schultz:

I feel quite quiet. . . . I am beginning to feel quite relaxed. . .
My ankles, my knees, and my hips feel heavy, relaxed, and
comfortable. . . . My solar plexus and the whole central portion of my body feel relaxed and quiet. . . . My hands, my arms,
and my shoulders feel heavy, relaxed, and comfortable. . . .
My neck, jaw, and my forehead feel relaxed, they feel comfortable and smooth. . . . My whole body feels quite, heavy, comfortable, and relaxed. . . . I am quite quiet. . . . My whole
body is relaxed, and my hands are warm and relaxed and warm,
my hands are warm, warmth is flowing into my hands, they are
warm, warm.

Patients may also increase their hand temperature by focusing
on images of the blood increasing into their hand.   During the
initial training period, patients are instructed that the speed at
which they elevate the hand temperature is more important than
the actual amount of degrees increased.   If the patient is able to

increase his hand temperature 1 to 2°F in 1 min at the first sign
of a headache, they may be successful in aborting an acute headache. At each session at the clinic, the biofeedback therapist
will review the patient's daily diary of practice sessions and
will also discuss which images the patient is using for the practice sessions.

The patient is weaned off the temperature trainer slowly. During
the final week of the initial training period, the patient is encouraged to practice, at home, twice daily on the machine and
twice daily without the monitor, using only the images which
have proven helpful for him. At this time, the patient is to touch
his hand or attempt to note any changes in his hands during a
practice session. Patients are not encouraged to purchase their
own temperature trainers as there is a tendency to rely on the
monitor rather than independent biofeedback techniques at the
first warning of a headache.

It is essential that the patient be encouraged to continue daily
practice sessions following the return of the temperature trainer.
Those patients who are faithful to a practice schedule will probably be able to continue to use these biofeedback techniques
successfully to abort headaches.

At each practice session at the clinic, the patient is monitored
on an EMG trainer for 20 min. The EMG electrodes are placed
on the frontalis muscle and the patient sits back in the recliner
chair. As the muscle relaxes, the tone of the EMG trainer will
decrease. The tone is usually highpitched and unpleasant in
order to encourage the patient to decrease it. At the initial session, the patient is given a set of progressive relaxation exercises adapted from the work of Joseph Wolpe. In these exercises, the patient is instructed to tense and relax the muscles
in the upper part of the body, helping him to identify which muscles are tense and giving him guidelines on relaxing these muscles. The exercises are as follows:

Let all your muscles go loose and heavy. . . . Just settle back
quietly and comfortably. . . . Wrinkle up your forehead now,
wrinkle it up tight; now smooth it out. . . . Picture your entire
forehead and scalp becoming smoother, as the relaxation increases and spreads. . . . Now frown and crease your brow;
study the tension. . . . Let go of the tension again, smooth out
your forehead once more. . . . Now, close your eyes tighter
and tighter; feel the tension. Now relax your eyes. . . . Keep
your eyes closed, gently, comfortably, and notice the relaxation
. . . . Now clench your jaws, bite your teeth together, study

the tension throughout your jaws. . . . Relax your jaws now;
let your lips part slightly; appreciate the relaxation. . . . Now
press your tongue hard against the roof of your mouth; look for
the tension. . . . Now let your tongue return to a comfortable
and relaxed position. . . . Now press your lips together, tighter
and tighter . . . Now relax your lips; notice the contrast between tension and relaxation. . . . Feel the relaxation all over
your face, all over your forehead and scalp, eyes, jaws, lips,
tongue, and your neck muscles. . . . Press your head back as
far as it can go and feel the tension in your neck. . . . Roll it
to the right and feel the tension shift. . . . Now roll it to the
left. . . . Straighten your head and bring it forward and press
your chin against your chest. . . . Now let your head return to
a comfortable relaxed position. . . . Study the relaxation. . . .
Let the relaxation develop. . . . Now shrug your shoulders tight,
right up. . . . Hold the tension, hold it . . . Now drop your
shoulders and feel the relaxation; neck and shoulders relaxed. .
. . Shrug your shoulders again and move them around. Bring
your shoulders up, forward and back. . . . Now let them relax
and feel the relaxation.

These exercises are to be used in home practice twice daily. If
the patient is also practicing temperature feedback training, he
is to use the progressive relaxation exercises following the 10
min on the temperature monitor. There is a tendency for the
hands to warm automatically while practicing the relaxation exercises, and if they are performed prior to the temperature
training session the hand temperature may be very high and the
practice session would be worthless.

Following the initial visit at the clinic, the progressive relaxation exercises are not completed while on the EMG monitor. In-
stead, the patient is advised to focus on relaxing the muscles in
the upper part of the body. Certain guidelines are given to the
patient to help him relax and decrease the tone of the monitor.
He is cautioned that sudden body or eye movements will sharply
increase the tone of the monitor. Also, swallowing or taking a
deep breath will affect the monitor. The patient is advised to
keep his mouth open partially if he is a teeth grinder or clenches
his jaws tightly. The tone may also decrease if he moves his
head forward, especially if he complains of neck tension.

The biofeedback therapist serves as a guide to the patient in identifying his stress points. It may be as simple as alerting him
that he is wrinkling his brows or tightening his shoulders. By
identifying and relaxing these stress points, many patients note
a decrease in the severity of their headaches. Patients may also

abort the acute headache by practicing the progressive relaxation exercises at the first sign of a headache.

Since many patients awaken with a headache, the patient is advised to practice immediately before bedtime. Portable EMG monitors are occasionally leased to a patient for home use when continuity of training is considered vital in helping him relax the stress points. Again, it is important to encourage continued daily practice at home. The patients who are most successful in using biofeedback training to decrease the frequency, severity, and duration of their headaches are usually diligent in their practice sessions. For out-of-town patients, returning home after the 2-week intensive period can decrease their abilities with biofeedback. While receiving the intensive biofeedback training, the patient is on a "therapeutic vacation" and free from the stresses of daily life. However, on the return to home and work, the problems are still there and the biofeedback training may be ignored. The patient must be encouraged and warned regarding this situation.

For all patients, incorporating the techniques of biofeedback training into everyday life is difficult. The biofeedback therapist and the physician must frequently encourage the patient to continue the daily practice and utilize these new techniques in combating the headache problem.

There are a variety of other techniques including hypnosis and those techniques espoused by followers of Zen, yoga, Transcendental Meditation, and other types of meditation and by physicians who use techniques of progressive relaxation. It does appear that some individuals who practice these techniques secure temporary relief from their tension states. However, in all these techniques the underlying factors that produce the tensions are not usually understood by the patient, so that rather than getting at the cause of the tension, a reconditioning or in some instances covering technique is used rather than insight and working through of the patient's problem.

References

1. W. Gowers: Diseases of the Nervous System, Vol. 2,
   Philadelphia, P. Blakiston Son & Company, 836-866,
   1893.

2. Definition of Migraine by the Research Group on Migraine
   and Headache. In: James W. Lance, Mechanism and
   Management of Headache, 4th Edition, Sydney, Butter-
   worth's, 1982.

3. Huckaday, J.M., Peet, K. M. S., and Huckaday, T. D. R.:
   Bromocriptine and migraine. Headache 16:109, 1976.

4. Couch, J. R., Ziegler, D. K., and Hassanein R.: Amitriptyline in the prophylaxis of migraine: Effectiveness in
   relationship of antimigraine and antidepressant drugs.
   Neurology 26:121, 1976.

5. Ekbom, K.: Lithium in the treatment of chronic cluster
   headache. Headache 17:39-40, 1977.

6. Jannetta, P.J.: Treatment of trigeminal neuralgia by
   suboccipital and transtentorial cranial operations. Clinical
   Neurosurgery 24:538-549, 1977.

7. Friedman, A. P., and Brenner, C.: Post-traumatic and
   histamine headache. Archives of Neurology and Psychiatry
   52:126, 1944.

8. Jacobson, S. A.: Mechanisms of the sequelae of minor
   craniocervical trauma. In: Walker, A. E., Cavens, W.
   F., and Critchley, M., eds. The Late Effects of Head
   Injury, Springfield, Illinois, Charles C Thomas Publishing,
   35-45, 1969.

9. Brenner, C., Friedman, A. P., Merritt, H. H., and
   Denny-Brown, D.: Posttraumatic headache. Journal
   of Neurosurgery 1:379, 1944.

10. Kay, D. W., Carrott, T. A., and Lassman, L. P.: Brain trauma in the postconcussional syndrome. Lancet, 1052-1055, November 13, 1971.

11. Sheeley, W. F.: Pre-existing disorder may underlie industrial psychiatric casualty. Clinical Psychiatry News 1:27-28, June, 1980.

12. Taylor, A. R.: Postconcussional sequelae. British Medical Journal 2:67, 1967.

13. Miller, H.: Accident neurosis. British Medical Journal 1:919, 922, 1961.

14. Critchley, M: In: Walker, A. E., Cavens, W. F., and Critchley, M., eds. The Late Effects of Head Injury, Springfield, Illinois. Charles C Thomas Publishing, 3, 1969.

15. Simon, D. J., and Wolff, H. G.: Studies on headache; Mechanism of chronic post-traumatic headache. Psychosomatic Medicine 8:227, 1946.

16. Haas, D. C., Pinada, G. S., and Lourie, H.: Juvenile head trauma syndromes and their relationship to migraine. Archives of Neurology 32:727-730, 1975.

17. Oldendorf, W. H.: Journal of Nuclear Medicine 3:382, 1962.

18. Vijayan, N., and Dreyfus, P. M.: Post-traumatic dysautonomic cephalalgia. Archives of Neurology 32:649-652, October, 1975.

19. Kelly, M.: Headaches: Traumatic and rheumatic. The cervical somatic lesion. Medical Journal of Australia 2:479, November 28, 1942.

20. Sargent, J. D., Green, E. E., and Walters, E. D.: The use of autogenic feedback training in a pilot study of migraine and tension headache. Headache 12:120-124, 1972.

21. Budzinsky, T., Stoyva, J., and Adler, C.: Feedback induced muscle relaxation application to tension headache. Behaviorial Therapy and Experimental Psychology 1:205, 1970.